Care at a Distance

Item due for return on or before the last date shown below		

D1355555

CARE & WELFARE

Care and welfare are changing rapidly in contemporary welfare states. The *Care & Welfare* series publishes studies on changing relationships between citizens and professionals, on care and welfare governance, on identity politics in the context of these welfare state transformations, and on ethical topics. It will inspire international academic and political debate by developing and reflecting upon theories of (health) care and welfare through detailed national case studies and/or international comparisons. This series will offer new insights into the interdisciplinary theory of care and welfare and its practices.

SERIES EDITORS

Jan Willem Duyvendak, University of Amsterdam
Trudie Knijn, Utrecht University
Monique Kremer, Netherlands Scientific Council for Government Policy
  (Wetenschappelijke Raad voor het Regeringsbeleid – WRR)
Margo Trappenburg, Utrecht University, University of Amsterdam

PREVIOUSLY PUBLISHED

Jan Willem Duyvendak, Trudie Knijn and Monique Kremer (eds.): *Policy, People, and the New Professional. De-professionalisation and Re-professionalisation in Care and Welfare*, 2006
  ISBN 978 90 5356 885 9
Ine Van Hoyweghen: *Risks in the Making. Travels in Life Insurance and Genetics*, 2007
  ISBN 978 90 5356 927 6
Anne-Mei The: *In Death's Waiting Room. Living and Dying with Dementia in a Multicultural Society*, 2008
  ISBN 978 90 5356 077 8
Barbara Da Roit: *Strategies of Care. Changing Elderly Care in Italy and the Netherlands*, 2010
  ISBN 978 90 8964 224 0
Janet Newman and Evelien Tonkens (eds.): *Participation, Responsibility and Choice. Summoning the Active Citizen in Western European Welfare States*, 2011
  ISBN 978 90 8964 275 2
Patricia C. Henderson: *AIDS, Intimacy and Care in Rural KwaZulu-Natal. A Kinship of Bones*, 2011
  ISBN 978 90 8964 359 9

CARE AT A DISTANCE

On the Closeness of Technology

Jeannette Pols

AMSTERDAM UNIVERSITY PRESS

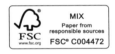

Cover photo: Ruud Mast

Cover design: Sabine Mannel, NEON graphic design company, Amsterdam
Lay-out: JAPES, Amsterdam

ISBN   978 90 8964 397 1
e-ISBN 978 90 4851 301 7 (pdf)
e-ISBN 978 90 4851 629 2 (ePub)
NUR   882

Contents

Part II Knowledge and promises

Part III Routines and efficiencies

Conclusions: On studying innovation

Nightmares, promises and efficiencies in care and research

1 Introduction

The telecare hype

'Telecare' is an umbrella term referring to the technical devices and professional practices applied in 'care at a distance', care that supports chronically ill people living at home.[1] With telecare, the formal or informal carer is not in the same place as the person receiving care. Instead, carers use new communication tools such as webcams, electronic monitors, email and websites to interact with patients, transmit data and provide instruction. Strictly speaking, the telephone is also a distant-care device and it is often central to making telecare practices work. The term telecare, however, commonly refers to the *new* technical arrangements for care or, as the critics might say, to a new hype in care.[2]

Hype is indeed a part of the introduction of telecare in health care. Innovations in telecare have seen optimists and pessimists hurrying onto the soapbox to proclaim their opposing views. Innovative practices are by definition not well researched, and these soapbox speeches emphasise either their pros – the promises telecare is bound to fulfil – or their cons, the nightmares it will inevitably bring.[3, 4, 5, 6]

The promises heard most often in the Netherlands, where the research reported in this book took place, concern improvements in efficiency.[7] Telecare promises to support care for a rapidly ageing population, when fewer younger people will be available to care for a rising number of older people with chronic diseases. This will have an even greater effect because telecare promises professional long-distance carers reciprocal support from their patients. Decision makers portray modern patients as active, eager and well able to care for themselves.[8] They claim that telecare will help patients manage their own care even better. In addition to claims for the more efficient use of personnel capacity, there is a very different efficiency promise: telecare will reduce the *cost* of health care.[9] Both types of efficiency alternate in telecare proclamations (see Chapter 7).

The inevitable nightmares, on the other hand, are full of grim images of care turned cold. Older people, instead of moving into a care institution when their minds and bodies start to fail, will have to stay at home, surrounded by all kinds of cold mechanical devices, receiving no support from caring people. Carers of these alienated people will only discover that someone has passed away when the sensors stop reporting movement and vital signs. Professionals, often nurses, lie awake, imagining the fate of neglected patients and overlooking serious problems because nobody actually bothers to go out and see these vulnerable patients any more.[10]

These polarised views are not so much a debate but a juxtaposition, a contest between 'inevitable' futures. Opponents accuse each other of either standing in the way of a desirable future, or of helping a horrific one emerge. The optimists accuse the pessimists of irrational resistance to obvious improvements and a shocking neglect of the best interests of patients. The pessimists accuse the optimists of trying to push technology that is not evidence-based down their throats[11] and, indeed, a shocking neglect of what is best for patients.

The debate is further troubled because telecare equipment comes in many shapes and sizes, from webcams to monitoring devices. The various items are often lumped together as 'telecare' in these debates, as if they all do the same thing. 'Smart home' devices such as sensors or alarms are sometimes included, as these devices support homecare processes or watch over vulnerable people.[12] Others sometimes throw in telemedicine devices as well, which are devices used for contact between professionals and their organisations.

The many potential users of the technologies, including patients, professionals, health care organisations, the industry and the families of the patients – all having their different hopes and concerns – cause even further clouding. And who is to pay the bill? Industries, care organisations, health insurers and the national government all point at each other to pay for the costly telecare infrastructure that has to be built. The Dutch government has structured national health care as a (regulated) market. This means that the government is 'pro' telecare, but it does not actively steer telecare development, although it does pay for screen-to-screen contact, and project organisers may opt for starter's grants.[13] The Dutch government wants care organisations, professionals, patient organisations and insurance companies to develop telecare projects together.

The producers of telecare devices are also involved, having an obvious interest in selling their devices and services. Much to their dismay, they cannot sell their products directly to patients, but must negotiate sales with professionals and often find the latter not all that interested. Although to date the Dutch national patient organisation is 'pro', the people who actually have to live with the devices have no voice (or choice) in the matter until their care providers offer them a particular telecare device.[14] Since the implementation of telecare is often done through pilot projects, such offers may come and go.[15]

Lack of knowledge

Clearly, there are two conflicting scenarios for the future of telecare and a confusing crowd of actively involved or mildly interested parties. Neither scenario – promise or nightmare – can be confirmed, rejected or modified yet. The telecare market does not seem to be selling many telecare products, and there have been some spectacular bankruptcies in projects and organisations already. Since there is no knowledge about the actual workings of telecare, the audience gathered round the soapbox will have to share the speaker's convictions or has to believe the story at face value.

This lack of knowledge may seem paradoxical, because international publications of studies evaluating individual telecare projects keep piling up. Yet these studies have not been able to substantiate the promises or deal with the worries. How can we understand this paradox? Mostly these studies reveal the difficulty of designing and conducting useful evaluation studies on complex care practices.[16] This has to do with the nature of the innovative care practices, the design and rationale of these studies, and the misfit between them.

Scientists model classic evaluation studies on the gold standard of research into the effectivity of interventions: the randomised controlled trial (RCT). The design of an RCT has strict conditions.[17] Researchers developed RCTs to test the effectivity of therapies, particularly drugs. RCTs create controlled conditions to observe how a relatively small number of variables changes value under the influence of a small number of other variables. To control conditions means setting up a control group of patients who do not receive the experimental therapy. The design averages out disturbing variables such as irrelevant differences between individual patients by assigning patients randomly to either the experimental or the control group. Preferably, both researchers and research subjects do not know to which group the patients are assigned. This is known as double-blind research. The research needs a substantial number of test persons for reliable comparisons and conclusions. The exact number depends on the number of variables to measure, the homogeneity of the test population, the threshold deemed acceptable for false positives or false negatives, and so on.

The strict requirements of RCTs can rarely be met when this research model is used on (tele)care practices. Randomisation is often impossible in small pilot projects, or it is ethically dubious. Carers and patients tinker with the telecare devices to make them fit to their purposes. Small pilot projects rarely engage a sufficient number of patients. For these reasons, many evaluations use suboptimal designs from the viewpoint of authoritative quantitative research.[18]

Another complication for conducting controlled studies in care practices is that it is hard to keep interventions stable. Telecare devices are not just interventions in the lives of individual patients, they intervene in care practices as well. When devices enter health care, established practices must be organised differently in order to fit in the new devices.[19] Consequently, nurses and patients may put the same devices to work in different ways in different places, thereby varying the actual intervention. For example, patients can use monitoring devices alone, assembling and interpreting the parameters themselves, or nurses may interpret the figures the patients produce in order to keep an eye on their shifting symptoms. The results of the research may thus be the outcome of varying interventions, even if they all use the same device. Rather than going to great lengths to report how and in which context people used the telecare devices in the study, researchers tend to describe interventions briefly in the method sections. Because researchers assume that specificities of the context are disturbing variables and average them out, differences rarely become transparent. The results remain local and as a result difficult to interpret, replicate and generalise.[20]

A related complication troubles research in innovative practices in particular. Quantitative research needs to work with the outcome variables defined at the start of the study. This book demonstrates, however, that innovative care practices are characterised by a process of identifying and adjusting goals, because participants are looking for ways to make new technologies work. In this process, the type of outcome is not fixed but participants are on the way to define them. How they do this is difficult to predict, particularly when there are many participants with different concerns and interests who all want to have things done their way. This implies that rather than proving the *effectivity* of predefined variables, it would be wiser to first articulate the various possible *effects* of using the new technology.[21]

Besides these methodological considerations, Dutch telecare practices demonstrate yet another problem with research peculiar to the Dutch health care market. The financing of telecare projects is often done in combination with the research undertaken to evaluate them. The industry, insurance company or care organisations thus own the results of the study and may publish them at will, or might decide to keep the results to themselves. Research results become business secrets that permit organisations to stay ahead of the competition. In technological innovation, business and research are often intertwined.[22]

Another twist in this entanglement of industries, health care organisations, financers and researchers is that telecare projects and their evaluation studies tend to start and end at the same time, regardless of the results. The research infrastructure keeps the telecare practice going, but also makes it fall apart when the research stops.[23] I will discuss the intricacies of research and telecare practices more extensively in the final chapter.

Noise and dust

Proponents and opponents of telecare innovations are making lots of noise, but at the same time, lots of dust clouds these innovations. It is simply unclear what telecare technology can achieve in care. Promises, nightmares, and dreams of efficiency have taken the place of knowledge and facts in the debate. Research data are inconclusive or belong to marketing departments rather than collective learning processes. Soapbox accusations are often angry harangues by worried parties. The type of telecare device and the funding depend on where you live in the Netherlands, on the organisation active locally, and on which devices they happen to have bought and managed to implement. Successful enterprise is the basis for implementation, not public consideration of what defines good care or a good life for individual patients, not knowledge about the workings of telecare. Developing telecare, then, is about clever networking and staying ahead of the competition rather than collective learning about the best form of care for whom.

This study

We do not know how telecare works, and market/soapbox policies for telecare development are not reassuring. The study in this book takes a different approach from soapbox speeches, market transactions, or the project evaluation study. It aims to develop a better way of thinking about technological innovations in care. Is it possible to develop reliable knowledge to support innovation? What would be useful to know? How could decision makers improve the process of telecare development?

To address these questions, I analyse and compare various pioneer telecare practices in the Netherlands, using an ethnographic approach to gain insight into how telecare changes health care. Ethnography is a good option compared to evaluation studies because it allows the researcher to ask open questions. It does not have to define outcome variables at the start of the research but takes these – the outcomes – as the result of the ethnographic study. It does not need large quantities of patients but may learn from small, pioneering practices. Ethnographic studies do not demand strict conditions for research, because they are developed to do research outside the laboratory.

Ethnographic studies analyse what new devices and people do as the *achievements* of practices rather than as points of departure. Researchers do not decide upon the outcome variables in advance, at the researcher's desk, but identify what is a key variable for understanding telecare practices *in situ*, from the practices in which people use telecare. What are the concerns in these practices? What values do people try to establish in care when they start using telecare? How do telecare devices shape these practices? I study telecare by *observing* how patients use it in their daily life practices and how professionals use it in their daily work practices. I *interview* those who work with telecare about their experiences, and ask the users to *observe their own practices*.

Ethnographic observation is never 'blank' registration. A theoretical understanding of the object of observation informs the observation as well as the registration. When people observe a flower, they immediately make assumptions about its plant-like characteristics. When the observer is a trained biologist, the plant-like characteristics can be refined further (the flower is a poppy, member of the family of Papaveraceae, its appearance points to the sour condition of the soil, and so on). This theorising or understanding is covert in the more commonsense observations of the world. In this study, I try to make them explicit by articulating[24] and then critically analysing the theories that shape our vision of care and technology.[25] For example, the theoretical assumption that technology *determines* what occurs in a situation is embedded in both the promises and nightmares articulated in the telecare debate.

To shape the ethnographic material, this study analyses theories of care and theories of technology as instruments or tools that help to perceive and articulate, to name and frame versions of the object under study.[26] What kind of 'things' are technologies supposed to be? How can we to interpret their workings? What does the text make readers think of the activity of caring? When is it good or bad?[27, 28] How do theories of care differ from observed care practices? Integrated in the ethnographic study, this theoretical analysis creates a set of instruments for naming and framing care and technologies that fits the observed care practices. Practices may correct existing theory and provide the building blocks for developing new theory. Using these tools, I articulate what (tele-)care is and what it becomes in specific daily life and work practices.

Three questions guide the analysis: What *normative shifts* in what participants regard as good can be witnessed when telecare devices enter care practices? What *types of knowledge* do various telecare devices bring into play? What *new routines* follow from the introduction of telecare, and what do these routines imply for what care becomes? Despite the inevitable intertwining of norms, knowledge and routines in care practices, I deal with these three questions separately in the three parts of the book. This differentiation serves to trace the various threads for the sake of the analysis, without suggesting they can or do exist separately.

In conclusion, I take up the question of how to think about technological innovation in care. I study how to improve the way innovative practices emerge, how people argue about them and make decisions about them. How can the process of innovation make better use of knowledge instead of relying on unsubstantiated promises or nightmarish threats?

Various telecare practices

This book contains ethnographic studies of various care practices. There is a telecare project in palliative care for oncology patients who will not recover from their disease. There are the webcams used by homecare organisations to provide professional support to people with severe lung disease (chronic obstructive pulmonary disease, COPD). These webcams also allow fellow patients in the homecare organisation to contact each other. There are the webcams used by professionals as a form of follow-up care when lung disease patients leave a rehabilitation clinic. In one project, call centre nurses monitor the vital signs (weight, blood pressure, pulse) of people with severe heart failure. These call centre nurses communicate with the nurses in the hospital, because the latter are responsible for the care of these patients. Another project has hospital nurses and heart failure patients using an educational device without the mediation of call centre nurses.

People with different chronic diseases use different devices. Telecare developers target people with a chronic disease most often, as they form the largest patient groups: COPD, heart failure, and diabetes. Palliative care is a new branch on the Dutch telecare tree. I introduce and discuss these telecare projects in the respective chapters. I list the complete collection of projects in the Appendix for the reader to look up if confusion threatens to strike. The scope of this book does not extend to telemedicine (technologically mediated communications between professionals) or smart home technology (technology working automatically in the home), and both have been excluded from the analysis.

Observing this variety of practices makes it clear that *care* takes place in various shapes and forms. It differs between people with different diseases, but also between configurations of patients, professionals and devices within the same patient group. Depending on the set-up, the possible role of the professional and the type of responsibility taken by the patient may differ dramatically. In telecare practices, participants are actively experimenting with new ways of shaping care. In this process, participants make implicit practices explicit, and what care is and how it should be becomes a matter of overt concern. This makes innovative telecare practices excellent places to learn about care. This concern runs throughout this book. I want to learn more about *what care is* by studying practices where precisely this question is at stake.

Studying innovative technologies

To study innovative and evolving practices I use tools developed from a material semiotic elaboration of domestication theory. Material semiotics stands for the idea that people and objects shape each other in mutual relations.[29] Identities are situated; they are the result of specific relations within a situation. For example, a person in a white coat using a stethoscope to listen to another person's heartbeat is most probably a doctor. The white coat and stethoscope help to create the 'doctor', but not by themselves. The characteristics of the person wearing the white coat, her working context and the patient's situation turn the using of a stethoscope into a doctor's activity rather than, say, a game or an act. The relation between humans and objects shape identities in practice, and these identities change when the practices, relations, and attributes change. The doctor from my example above may become a mother when she picks up her child from the local school.

My colleague Dick Willems and I missed this mutuality of adaptation – and thus the interdependence between technology and users – in both domestication and deterministic theories of technology.[30] We were looking for concepts that could make researchers sensitive to relationality, which is why we were interpreting domestication theory in material semiotic terms.[31] Domestication originally referred to the processes that led to humans living together with animals and plants, but this term has since been adapted to include technology in order to analyse how humans put technology to use. Domestication theory forms a counter story to deterministic understandings of technology, where the fate of a certain practice is at the mercy of the workings of a technology. Domestication theory granted humans more agency: animals, plants and technologies do not determine our lives but come to live with *us*, in our homes, and on our terms. This approach informed the study of creative use practices where users put technologies to different uses than their designers intended.

Humans put technology, animals, and plants to use, and allow them into their homes. To make this relational, one should look at the other parties, too. Animals, plants and technology also 'let' humans into their environment, or set the terms for living together with them. Nomadic people, for instance, follow their flocks. Other animals 'refuse' to live with humans, like the vicuñas in the Andes.[32] To exploit the precious wool of the vicuña, humans tried keeping them in captivity, but the vicuña almost became extinct in the attempt. The humans had to set the vicuñas free and had to follow them high into the mountains to harvest their wool. One could argue that the vicuñas 'set' the conditions for living with them.

Unlike vicuñas, technologies do not set their own terms by 'dying' from maltreatment, although they may get neglected to the point of 'social death'. However, new technologies such as telecare are still far from domesticated, a state that would be signified by more or less common, culture-bound practices of living or working together between humans and a certain 'species' of technology. Heuristically speaking, one can look for any of four – sometimes overlapping – activities that 'unleash' and 'tame' individuals and devices, which precedes the domestication of a species or their living together – or apart – happily ever after.

First, when new technology is 'let out of its box', individual devices are *unleashed* into the daily life practices to which they come to belong. This means that their actual effect and working are unpredictable. They can do all kinds of unexpected things. For instance, people domesticated the telephone quickly because it facilitated the social chatter of American women, even if its designers created it to transmit the business conversations of American men.[33] People domesticated the telephone, but differently than expected. The history of technology shows again and again that devices will behave differently to what their designers intended.

The second activity in the process of mutual adaptation involves *taming* the devices, in the sense that humans try to make them fit in with how they want to use them in practice. For example, few people use all the functions their personal computers provide; they just use the ones they need and know about. These unleashing and taming processes go the other way around as well. The third heuristic for analysing domestication processes looks at how devices unleash the imagination and creativity of their users who promptly invent new applications. This happens, for instance, when physicists or chemists put substances to new uses. Chapter 3 gives an example of how nurses in a heart failure clinic imagined different uses for telecare devices. They envisioned using them as research tools for their patient group, rather than for individual patient care, and explored the possibilities for adapting the devices for this purpose.

The fourth heuristic is to see how devices tame humans in their turn by allowing for, or even forcing, some activities while hindering others. A mundane example is the television that shows only ten channels instead of the 30 advertised in the TV guide. Some technologies are more coercive than others; a speed bump is coercive because it forces drivers to slow down to prevent damage to their cars.[34] Michel Foucault has analysed how the panopticon makes prisoners guard themselves; this exemplifies how objects can tame people into doing things.[35]

These four forms of unleashing and taming have heuristic value. Ultimately, it is often unclear who did what first to arrive at a certain collaboration. In the resulting practice, humans and devices have established their particular relations. Their identities and functions are interdependent. Unleashing and taming processes may lead to a fit between individual devices and users, and, eventually, to a form of domestication, implying more or less stabilised practices of cooperation, such as those of the telephone. These processes may also lead to the immediate or eventual rejection of a device (or, to be consistent, to a rejection of the humans), as happens with technology nobody wants to buy or to museum exhibits on the history of technology.

There are niche applications. For example, DJs still use vinyl records and turntables, which unleashed the invention of 'scratching', where the DJ moves a disc manually to produce the scratching sound. Also, stable practices may differ from one place to the next. For example, people use mobile phones differently in different places. As Donner points out:

> [The] widespread practice of 'beeping' between mobile phone users in sub-Saharan Africa [...] involves calling a number and hanging up before the mobile's owner can pick up the call. The mobile's call log and address book functions signal who called, and when. Most beeps are requests to the mobile owner to call back immediately, but beeps can also send a pre-negotiated instrumental message such as 'pick me up now', or send a relational sign, such as 'I'm thinking of you'. (Donner 2009)

The fit between humans and devices and the practices it leads to, for example, if the practice is a *caring* practice, is an empirical question. It demands careful analysis of the implemented routines, the stable or contentious norms and aims, and the issues addressed for solving.

To detect change, it is not enough to listen to the participants' accounts; people may take things and events for granted in daily life. Routine practices may (have) become invisible to participants, but may be visible to an involved observer. Devices obviously do not speak, and their doings can only be observed and spoken *about*. Detailed insight into what happens in care practices is thus important for learning what care actually means in a particular situation. This explains my partiality to ethnographic methods; they allow you to see people and devices 'in action', in the reciprocal taming and unleashing processes in the struggle for fit, even if the participants are unaware of what exactly changes along the way.

The chapters

Part one, 'Norms and nightmares', explores normativities in care and how they can shift when telecare is put to use. They deal with the nightmares of coldness and alienation in particular.

Chapter 2 studies a telecare project in palliative oncology. It analyses the normative opposition between warm care and cold technology. Warm care refers to good care for patients as subjects, whereas cold care refers to rational, technical medical care that relates to patients as objects. In the case study, however, the technology provided care that these theorists would label as warm. The study shows that metaphors of temperature are not particularly suitable for discerning good from bad care. I explore another concept for good care: *care that fits*.

Chapter 3 discusses the nurses' fear that telecare will impoverish patient care, because it could hinder the development of good relations with patients. Nurses also fear that telecare will make it harder for them to notice if patients have problems, because they are not actually visiting them at home. The chapter analyses how telecare changes the work practices of the nurses involved, and, with that, their notions of *good* care. Telecare challenges the idea that 'seeing the patient' is the gold standard for good nursing care, without dismissing the idea altogether. Contrary to expectation, telecare supported the nurses' desire to spot in time any troubles that patients might have. However, the *type* of problem changed. Neglected households became less important than a change in symptoms. Instead of making any sign relevant, telecare selected particular signs to look for and intensified their control. The concept of 'fit' from the first chapter gains more substance here. Fit not only refers to the relation between nurses and individual patients but also to notions of what is a problem and how best to care for that problem.

The second part, 'Knowledge and promises', discusses the implications of using telecare devices for the kind of knowledge that can be accessed, used and developed. I relate this analysis to the promise of increased self-management for chronic patients that telecare is supposed to provide.

Chapter 4 juxtaposes two ways of living with chronic disease incorporating telecare. Two devices help to shape the way each patient lives with their disease in important ways. The devices influence the understanding of what the problem is, what to do about it, who should do this, and what knowledge helps the person to do it. In doing so, the telecare practice intervened in or co-existed with other forms of care. A fit was not always established. Instead of one 'self' doing all the managing, various collectives set to work consisting of patients, professionals, family, friends, and devices, each implying different tasks and responsibilities for the participants. Patients were never caring for themselves 'alone'. Instead, the question was *who else* was involved in organising their care. Was there a key role for professionals, or did the patients undertake their own care together with friends, family, and fellow patients?

Chapter 5 analyses in more depth the relation between knowledge and the role of telecare technology. Instead of setting the patient's knowledge in opposition to the doctor's knowledge, the chapter contrasts scientific medical knowledge with the practical knowledge of patients. Patients use and develop practical knowledge that allows them to live their daily life with their disease. If the knowledge they receive – albeit embedded in devices or otherwise – is not practical or 'ready to use', they have to translate it to make it fit their situation, for better or for worse. They have to do this anew in every new situation. In the process of assembling, creating, and fitting practical knowledge, the patients enact their bodies in different ways. The question is how telecare may fit the use and development of practical knowledge.

The third part, 'Routines and efficiencies', analyses how telecare devices influence caring routines. The analysis unravels 'what's in a routine' in relation to the promise that telecare will bring efficiency.

Chapter 6 identifies the deeds of the webcam. What does it do? Users and scholars often praise the webcam as an intimate means of communication for care at a distance because of its invisibility and absence. It is a 'see-through device' that does not influence or hinder what is seen or said. However, I show how the webcam contributes to intimacy by its active presence rather than by its absence – for instance, by making people stare at each other's faces on the screen. The workings of the webcam delineate the limits of its use. As a means of communication, people may experience it as intrusive. Patients were reluctant to use webcams for contact with people they did not know. The proximity invoked by the webcam did not fit the distance demanded for relating to strangers.

Chapter 7 tackles the question of efficiency head on by analysing routines in care as forms of efficiency. Managers often take efficiency as a 'good in itself', of which there is only one variety, usually brought about by rationalisation and cost reduction. The chapter shows that efficiency itself cannot be a goal of care; efficiency comes in different versions that are fixed to particular versions of how the content of care is shaped. It is impossible to separate what (good) care comes to mean from the way in which it is organised. Changes in routines imply changes in the goals of care and in ways of defining the problems. It is always wise to question how claims of efficiency fit to what kind of care.

In the final chapter, I return to the question of how to understand innovation in care. My analyses suggest new ways of studying innovation, ways that fit better with the way care practices work and with the normativity embedded in care practices, and that make better use of knowledge about the workings of telecare technologies.

PART I

Norms and nightmares

2 Caring devices

About warm hands, cold technology and making things fit

Warm care, cold technologies

Theorists of medicine as well as lay people often put healthcare technology, including telecare, in opposition to warm human care and contact. They assume that medical technology is cold, rational and functional, whereas human care is affective and comforting. Where does this opposition of warm and cold care come from? Social theorists often distinguish care from biomedicine and management, presenting the latter as examples of the Habermassian system world. This system world has a logic of instrumentality and threatens to colonise the 'life world' characterised by intersubjective relations.[1] Opposing biomedicine and care in the trope of 'system world conquers life world' makes a spatial contrast. On the one hand, there are biomedical practices dominated by technical, objectifying and causal reasoning about the body and its diseases. On the other hand, warm care occurs between people, and patient subjectivity flourishes in the empathic relations between carer and patient at home. Warm care relates to sensitivity and concern, to 'being there' for those in need.

Although theorists accept that there is a legitimate space for detached and objectified medical treatment, for instance, in setting the proverbial broken bone, the opposition of warm and cold is partial to warmth. The metaphors criticise instrumental and objectifying treatments by pointing to the concern for the shivering patient needing a warm blanket after the bone-setting operation. Although necessary, the operation is a cold technical intervention, whereas the blanket signifies warm care and thus makes the practice 'good'. Warmth, then, equals goodness.[2]

Ironically, theorists often interpret the work of Michel Foucault, the philosopher who so subtly analysed the advent of clinical knowledge, as critical of medical rationality.[3] David Armstrong (1983), for instance, interprets Foucault's analyses as conceiving all medical knowledge as a form of discipline or surveillance.[4] People start regarding themselves and others with a monolithic, totalitarian medical gaze. For these Foucault interpreters, subjectivity is not merely oppressed but is invaded and shaped by a medical logic that disciplines the ways individuals behave and perceive themselves. Without being aware of it, people reshape themselves according to medical norms.

In the opposition between warmth and coldness, or care and medicine, technology is especially cold.[5] The philosophy of technology further enforces dichotomies between technical objects and affective subjects. A Heideggerian inheritance has taken root in commonsense thinking about what technology does. Technology gets 'in between' us and the world, alienating us from natural, unmediated ways of relating to what is around us.[6] Medical technology has a rational and functional image.[7] Devices may be clumsy and ugly, but they do what they have to do and are not regarded as part of a person's life world, although the industry is busy changing this.[8, 9, 10]

Warm and cold care stand for a more broadly defined opposition that separates an *ethical* relation to patients from an *epistemological* relation to patients. In an ethical relation, the clinician is empathic and involved and tries to care for patients as persons who have perspectives of their own, have feelings about their situation and concerns that encompass more than their disease. In an epistemological relation, the clinician is detached, like a scientist, and attempts to objectify what is the state of the patient's body, interferes in it and evaluates the result. In this chapter, I empirically question the metaphors of warmth and coldness and the oppositions they stand for. To make this as concrete as possible, I take some of the worries about cold care by technologies as a starting point and proceed with an empirical analysis of the workings of a specific tele-care device.

What (un)makes a human?

When framing technology as 'cold', a central fear is that it will replace humans and face-to-face contact.[11] The fear is that those already deprived of social contact will lose even more when technology takes over the tasks done by humans.[12] The horror image is the alienated old woman, detached from the world, surrounded by machines. This is the first objection Sparrow & Sparrow formulate in their 2006 paper on the use of robots in care for older people. Sparrow & Sparrow carefully consider whether robots could take over caring tasks from humans without losing quality of care. Their firmly negative answer resonates with the fear of dehumanisation.[13] Their arguments articulate the suspicion, deeply rooted in Western experience, of using machines in care.

Apart from the fear that technology will dehumanise care, Sparrow & Sparrow have at least three other objections against technical care. The first is that machines do not improve *control* because of their limited functionality. They can only perform specific tasks and will not help fulfil alternative needs. The second argument is that machines do not really care for us and certainly *do not love us*. Machines cannot have feelings or express empathy. The premise is that no person can feel cared for without being on the receiving end of real affection and concern. Robots and machines can only take over the instrumental – cold – parts of care.[14]

Finally, Sparrow & Sparrow warn that technology cannot relate *individually* to humans. Technology is predictable and standardised to perform one simple trick rather than another. People can switch it off at will, and it lacks the characteristics that make people care for other people – and pets – who have unpredictable needs that may call for attention at odd times.[15] Good relations take other people as 'ends in themselves', not as a means to something else. You cannot achieve this, Sparrow & Sparrow argue, when the other can be 'switched off or put on pause' and is consequently completely dependent on our own manipulations.[16]

Table 1 Why technology is cold

Technology...
does not enhance control
takes the place of human relations
has no feelings and so, cannot love us
cannot relate individually to humans

Based on Sparrow & Sparrow, 2006

Palliative care in Friesland

How does this image of cold technology relate to telecare practice? I studied care in a practice people generally think that warmth is the primary ingredient: palliative care. Palliative care is for those ill people whom doctors cannot cure. Professionals support patients to allow them the best possible quality and duration of life.[17] In the northern Dutch province of Friesland, the location of the project studied, professionals were concerned about a particular group of their incurably ill cancer patients. The disease can cause severe complaints, especially pain. The patients were on chemotherapy, not with the intention of curing their disease but to help keep tumours at bay and reduce their impact on their condition and remaining years of life. Chemotherapy can cause distressing side effects, such as fever, nausea, vomiting, constipation, loss of hair, ruined mucous membranes, and so on. Most symptoms can be effectively treated or tended, but, as the hospital staff in Friesland learned, these patients tended to underreport their complaints and suffer in silence. The project intended to reach out to these all too silent patients in order to treat them more adequately. To this end, they brought in a communication device called the health buddy or 'white box', the patients' own name for the device.

The white box is a telecommunication modem installed in the patient's home (see Illustration 1). It transmits data over the telephone line to a server that encodes them, and then on to a personal computer in the oncology department of the hospital. Every day the patients receive a list of questions that they answer by pressing the blue buttons. A flashing light indicates that the new questions have arrived for the day. The list starts with an extensive check of symptoms and continues with questions on psychosocial well-being, spiritual questions on coping with imminent death, information about diet, and so on. A team of medical professionals and the project coordinator from the company that distributes and maintains the white boxes developed the question protocol, which is the same for all patients. The session ends with a 'quote of the day', wisdom borrowed from classical and popular philosophers.

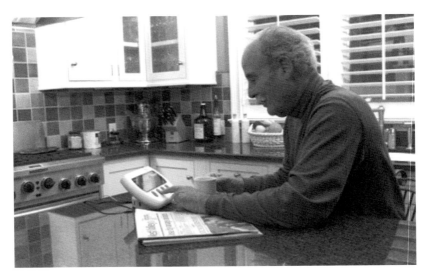

Illustration 1 Using the white box

The software in the server automatically codes answers with a red flag whenever patients may need specialist intervention – for instance, if the patient reports fever. It also flags cases more difficult to interpret, such as alarming answers to the questions on spiritual and psychosocial well-being. When flagging an answer, the white box gives patients feedback, urging them to call the nurse, adding the telephone number. In any event, each session reminds patients that they can always call the nurse or their GP. If they do not call, the nurse may respond to the alarm and call a patient to discuss if she needs to do something.

Clearly, designers did not intend the white box to be cold, merely functional technology. The white box aims to tend to psychological, social, physical and spiritual matters and acknowledges the subjectivity of patients in their struggle with disease rather than just dealing with their medical condition. However, you could argue that providing spiritual care through technology takes away humanity and intimacy. Compared to the ideal of discussing such matters in person, telecare communication may be seen as second best, with the patient at home, alone, answering hard questions outside the context of human(e) conversation, immediate attention and a supportive hand on the shoulder. In this interpretation, telecare swaps human care for technological attention.

However, this is not what the patients and their families reported when I visited them.[18] Patients and spouses were eager to convince me that they felt extremely well cared for. One couple used a Dutch idiom for luxury: they felt 'bedded on cotton wool' [*in de watten gelegd*]. This is a metaphor for softness rather than warmth, but it shows the patient's satisfaction with the device. How did care achieve this? One explanation is that patients did not regard the telecare system as a 'separate' thing in their care but as part of all the care they were getting, which they were especially pleased to receive. General appreciation was certainly there, but, as I will demonstrate, this is not the whole story. The telecare system made a specific contribution in the caring arrangements. The questions I ask in this chapter are: how do the participants and the telecare system re-shape care, and what does this say about the opposition between 'warm care' and 'cold technology'?

Situating matters of disease

Let me start with some background on the patients' situation. My informants reported that learning their diagnosis was a devastating experience. It was a 'bomb' falling down on their world, or a 'blow to the head'. The impact was a telling image of a barren battlefield or a blanked out perception, instead of normal life following its predictable course. Whatever had seemed clear and straightforward in life was no longer that. Loss of certainty and control and lots of empty spaces and questions confronted people. What will happen? How will I react to chemotherapy? What does it mean now that death is, somehow, coming closer? What will happen to my partner and kids?

> Mrs Jansen:[19] When they told me, the diagnosis hit me like a bomb. I didn't feel ill. I was functioning like I always did. A little pain here [points to her belly], but just *slight*. And then this diagnosis. You don't have a clue what's going to happen to you.

The chaos created by the diagnosis creates a demand for information, facts, predictions and new footholds. Patients have to establish a new order to enable a life with a completely changed perspective. As the oncology nurse told me: 'We are all immortal, until we fall ill,' meaning that we do not or are unable to reckon with death before the circumstances actually force us to do so. The patient, however, was not the only one taking the blow and experiencing a loss of control. The illness inflicted family, friends and neighbours, too. Sometimes patients stated that their family had more trouble dealing with the new situation than they had.

> Mrs Hallenforder: The first 14 days it was just... he [her husband] couldn't speak, he couldn't eat, couldn't sleep anymore. *I* have the disease, but he avoided everyone, talked to no one. Later my son told me: 'We [he and his father] didn't look at each other, the first 14 days. We stood there in the stable, milking the cows with our backs turned. We couldn't look each other in the face because then we would have started crying.'

Those who receive the prognosis that they or their loved ones would not recover from the disease needed a new order, but too many 'reminders' were unproductive. The patients did not want to be struck down repeatedly by having their situation pointed out to them again and again. Somehow, daily life with all its minor ups and downs and trivial developments had to continue, for as long as it could. It is good when a device reminds one of one's disease, but it is also good not to dwell upon it. Mr Frederiks worked in a shop when he fell ill:

> They [the customers] constantly wanted to know what was going on, how you are, really, right down to the bone. But if you tell that story 10, 20, 30 times a day, you get sick of being ill. That's really heavy, psychologically speaking. So I said: 'If you want to visit a patient, come when I'm in hospital having chemo.' Tube stuck into my hand, me lying flat out on a bed, nurse in the vicinity. Then I'm sick. Not on other days. Outside the hospital I don't want to be confronted by this. Then it'd rule your life. I don't want to be just someone sick. That's not how I want to live my life.

It is important to care for one's illness, but it is impossible to be a sick person all day and have one's identity and concerns narrowed down to the illness. My informants told me it was crucial to continue with ordinary life and keep up their interest in other people. They reconsidered their priorities and often spent more time with their loved ones. Still, they were very much aware of the illness: 'It's always there. When you wake up, you think, gosh, I have cancer. It's never not there, device or not.' The *presence* of the disease was a given, but not the scale, shape or understanding of it.

So there were at least two, sometimes conflicting demands on care for these patients. On the one hand, care had to provide handholds for dealing with the disease, the palliative chemo treatment, and ways of dealing with physical deterioration and approaching death, both for the patients and those living around them. On the other hand, the environment could not supply handholds too often, as that would make life unbearable. It is impossible to be an incurably ill person who is dying all day long; it would be impossible to continue showing an interest in the everyday muddle of ongoing life. In this field of tensions the telecare system played its part.

How did the patients and the telecare system shape the process of caring here? The exchange of content through the white box helped patients find a 'new order' in the chaos brought about by their new situation, but not merely that. The very *presence* of the device, the *regularity* of its demands for attention, the *modest investment of time* needed to complete the questionnaire and the *repetitiveness* of the questions all contributed to the creation of order.

> Mr Frederiks: It's a bit of self-discipline. It makes you aware of certain things. Have I got fever, did I throw up, have I weighed myself? I always do what the white box tells me to do. It says: 'Did you step on the scales today?' so I go to the scales and check my weight. I do the questions, and when I am done with the white box, I concentrate on the rest of my day. It is a moment of checking. I send information to the hospital, and get some information back for me. That's what the white box does for me.

Every day the light on the white box flashes to signal the arrival of new questions. Taking the time to answer the questions made Mr Frederiks think about his illness and how he felt, reminding him to care for himself and his disease. That is what he meant by his 'discipline'. The white box made him ask himself 'How am I today?' in comparison to the day before. The device made him analyse and articulate how he was doing, and made him take specific action. It only took a few minutes and allowed him to continue with whatever else he wanted to do afterwards. Thus, the illness received a designated place in his daily life, connected to his use of the white box. It was his *memento mori*, or at least 'remember caring', after which he went on with his day.

So while the telecare system helped to create and manipulate *time* for disease, it also created *space* for matters concerning disease. Technicians often installed the white box in the living room, because this is where most people have their telephone connection. It was not placed in the centre of the room, but often near a table where patients, with or without companions, could sit down to think about and answer the questions. Patients could spare their visitors a long list of complaints, having dealt with them on the white box.

> Mrs Fransen: You answer questions every day, and that's how you let them know if something is wrong. And when someone visits, I'm glad and don't feel the need to complain about how bad I feel. So, it's a nice alternative. It helps. You don't have to wait for somebody to show up.

The regularity and position of the white box helped to tame disease matters, and also helped to create time and space for an ordinary life as well.

Having an incurable disease and facing death is as terrible as it is abstract. By helping to ground disease matters, the device met the criterion of control that Sparrow & Sparrow formulated for good care: it gave the users a sense of control over their lives by allowing them to situate matters of disease and dying in time and space, even if this did not work for everyone (more on this below). This includes warm care qualities in the workings of the technology. The device helped patients deal with emotions and provided support. However, there were also elements from the cold side, such as the list of symptoms. The device could support more detachment in routine tasks such as weighing oneself. It put a boundary on self-pity or empathy from one's spouse: five minutes a day might be just enough. The patients used comparative expressions related to space, time, order and size. These terms provide criteria for shaping *the right scale* for matters to do with illness and care (not too much, not too little). The categories run through the dichotomies of coldness and warmth, opening up a different set of concerns.

Building relations through the white box

Sparrow & Sparrow's greatest worry, the most prominent commonsense fear of technology, is that machines will replace all human contact, making care cold by reducing it to mechanical interactions with machines. My informants, however, reported something else. They pointed to the ability of the telecare system to *bring people together*. Particularly patients living with partners reported that the questions on the white box gave them openings to discuss difficult subjects, or to reflect on how they had been doing in the past.

> Mrs Torensen: Well, he [her late husband] did the symptom checks really fast, hop, hop, hop, just like that. Then, the other questions, sometimes we'd sit down and talk about them. We'd be thinking, this is a kind of communication that we wouldn't have that often together. The white box hands you, say, a problem. And then you can talk to each other about it. That's really good, I really enjoyed that. It would bring up subjects that are not so easy to talk about. For instance, it asks if you can talk about things with your children. The box asks about something, you talk about it and it makes you think: how *do* we discuss this with the children? And that brings you to quite different conversations, really.

Instead of severing ties, the technology seemed to strengthen bonds by making people talk about subjects other than day-to-day matters. Besides handing them topics to discuss, the white box gave the informants the *language* in which they could talk about disease matters.

Mrs Torensen: You see, Gerald emailed friends and family, and so on. When he'd had chemo, he would email them about how his week had been, and so on. And I noticed that as time went by, he became far more open in his emails to others. And I still think that is because he had to name it, each time, how he felt, what was going on. I feel that it may help people get past the barrier of being close-mouthed. He could not only tell people that he'd been ill, but also how ill he'd been.

Mr Torensen had learned to articulate how he was doing, and this helped him stay in touch with his family and relatives. The white box literally provided him with words (better than yesterday, worst than last time, particular symptoms showing strongly, mildly or not at all). It had opened him up.

Apart from connecting patients to their loved ones, the white box also linked the patients to the nurse. The telecare system functioned as a new communication line to her. One message the system got across clearly to all informants was this: 'Please call the oncology nurse when there is trouble. You can never call us too much, you can only call us too little.' The nurse who called patients if she thought contact was needed only reinforced the importance of calling. The white box helped to establish an easily accessible phone connection between patient and nurse.

Mr Smit: It is really nice to know that you can call the oncologist [nurse] directly. It makes it all closer.
Mrs Smit/patient: There is less of a threshold, each time they tell you: 'Call the oncologist, here's the phone number, otherwise call your GP.' Here they don't give a phone number, because it's different for everyone. So the message is clear: 'Call, call, call. Don't be shy. Call.' So that gets you going, too.

In general, the connection between nurse and patient was probably the most successful achievement of the telecare system. All patients reported this. With the white box, the telecare system managed to establish and strengthen human relations rather than disrupt or replace them.

When human relations are warm, the telecare system, again, provides warm care. But do human relations always guarantee warmth? The patients also talked about relations that came undone when they fell ill. They gave quite a few examples of friends or family who walked out on them because they did not want to confront illness and death. The literature propagating warm care overflows with critical examples of uncaring professionals. Warm care needs *good* relations. The telecare system supported good relations by strengthening ties that were already good. This is why the patients saw the white box as a warm and caring technology.

On the other hand, the warm contact with the nurse mostly served to deal with 'cold' matters, such as medication and pain relief. Treatment of symptoms was the most important reason for both nurse and patient to get in touch.

Mrs Dodijn: She [the nurse] called me later in the day, and I asked why. She said a red flag had come up for my dizziness [Mrs Dodijn had reported a high degree of dizziness]. She wanted to know what had caused it. Well, I knew! From vomiting after chemo. I was so sick, so nauseous, I couldn't keep anything down. So I thought: that's why I'm dizzy. So she said: Let's handle this another way. I'll ask the doctor to give you more pills for the nausea. So I had one and three [pills], but now I have two, three and four, plus two extra. And now, the two extra make me constipated.

One could label Mrs Dodijn's nausea, dizziness, vomiting, tablets and constipation as 'cold' matters. It is also clear, however, that in this situation it is necessary to deal with cold matters to craft good care. Setting warm versus cold, good versus bad, subjective versus objective is problematic. Rather than opposing an ethical relation between subjects or an epistemological relation between subject and object, it seems that the creation of a *practical and aesthetic relation of making something fit* needs *both* ideas. This may be a better way of thinking about good care, to include elements formerly dubbed cold. Caring is good when it seeks to fit the situation of the individual patient, as in 'tailor-made care'. Nausea, dizziness or family relationships may trouble some people sometimes, but not others. Good care needs both subjective and objective elements, mixed to different tastes and concerns, depending on the situation at hand.

Devices do not love us

What does the analysis of the workings of the telecare system reveal about the notion of 'fitting'? Sparrow & Sparrow made it clear that you cannot expect a device to 'love' you. Inanimate devices obviously do not have feelings. However, expressions of love and concern for others did become apparent in two forms: as care for the nurse and as care for the device. Primarily, the patients experienced using the device as a way of caring for the nurse. This has nothing to do with actual love *by* devices, as Sparrow & Sparrow rightly show is impossible, but with expressing concern *through* devices.

Mr Dieriks: You have this thing [white box] that makes it easy to pass information on to the nurse. The step to fill out the questions is far easier than phoning the nurse or a doctor. You know these people are busy, they have patients, meetings. You always feel, if you call, you'd only be disturbing. I don't have that with the white box. They can read it when it suits them and I've still passed on my information. That's nice.

Mr Dieriks does not want to disturb the nurse, but more than that, he is willing to *help the nurse and doctor care for him*. The telecare system provides a device that aligns the demands of not wanting to disturb, responding responsibly to problems when they appear, and helping to care for the professionals in return. Thus, the white box is a device that helps patients to actively care for their nurses just as much as the other way around. Mrs Smit became aware of her own caring role the time she did not report how unwell she was feeling.

> Mrs Smit: I'd had the flu, and then got really bad anaemia. I couldn't get warm. Well, we survived the weekend, no problem. Then she [the nurse] called about something to do with the device and heard that I was in bed, shivering. She can't see that through the device! She couldn't have known I was unwell from the questions. I'd called my GP for antibiotics, for the flu. And I went to the hospital on Monday for another course of chemo and she said: 'O my God, I didn't know.' She was shocked when she saw me.
> Mr Smit: We should have called [about your flu], really.
> Mrs Smit: Yes, it was a mistake not to call. Because it meant they didn't know what was happening to me.
> Mr Smit: You have to learn this.

What Mr and Mrs Smit had to learn was that reporting complaints was not just a matter of *bothering* professionals with things unimportant, but of *helping* them to plan their treatment. When Mrs Smit, a particularly thin 76-year-old, showed up shivering from anaemia, she could not get the planned course of chemotherapy and got a blood transfusion instead. But there was also the matter of the upset nurse: the patient was so ill, and the nurse was shocked to realise that neither she nor the telecare system had noticed. This turn of events made the patient feel as if she had 'made a mistake' by not reporting her bad condition.

So 'helping the nurse' was a strong motivation for using the white box and reporting complaints, and this gave the patients support in return: they were happy to help and act like 'good patients'.

Then there was the *love for the device*. The white box took the initiative by demanding the patient's help. The patients cared for the box because it told them what they could do to help. The following quote shows this reversal of roles, with the patient caring for the device instead of the other way around.

> Mr Klaasen: Well, I'm not usually in a rush to phone, and now you don't even have to call. [laughs] That's the benefit. I'm not one for telling long tales on the phone. But then I think: Hey, here he is again, *that buddy wants to ask me something*. It's become more or less a friend of mine, so to speak. It's like you have a cat or a little dog. I have my health buddy. [emphasis mine, JP]

The white box does not put the patient in the position of having to ask busy doctors or nurses for help: the buddy asks Mr Klaasen questions, and he is happy to oblige. Addressing the white box as a friend or pet also points to how the white box has itself become an 'end' rather than a 'means' for Mr Klaasen. He was happy with the device for being there and keeping him company. It exemplifies a caring relation between human and device.

Love for the device and care for and from the nurse can also become entangled.

> Mrs Wilkens: I think it is really great. We always say: here's Tania [nurse] winking again. You see, when the light starts flashing [to announce the arrival of questions], we say: Tania is winking at us.

Here, the white box is a metonym for the nurse, signifying her presence and the care and support she provides – with a little help from the patient. If anything, the use of the device does not put care at a distance but in close proximity, since it facilitates closer and more frequent contact with the professional carers in the hospital.

These examples show the different roles of patients who care for nurses and devices, as compared to nurses and devices caring for patients. For the *nurse*, affection is not the sole part of a good professional caring relationship. The nurse may appreciate her patients, she may understand them and be empathic, she may even like them, but she does not *love* them, nor is this necessary or desirable for her care to be good. She should bring in her knowledge of symptoms and cures, ways of dealing with nausea and pain, and the ability to judge what is relevant for individual patients. This would be called 'cold care' in the warm-cold dichotomy, but the term sounds awkward here.

On the other hand, patients can be far more liberal with love. They may love the device and care for the nurse, but they can only do this because the device and the nurse look after the knowledge aspect of the caring relationship. Patients depend on this knowledge that they do not possess themselves. What they offer is 'material' that helps the nurses build their clinical picture – and their appreciation for the accuracy of their diagnosis and treatment. To call a professional caring relationship good, it indeed needs some of the presumably cold characteristics: knowledge of symptoms and their treatment, experience of patients with comparable forms of cancer, the ability to discern worries from symptoms, the capacity to behave and react appropriately, and so on.

Professional care, by both humans and machines, can be analysed more adequately in terms of continuously shaping a match between needs and interventions. In terms of the aesthetics of fit, both warm and cold elements are present, as long as their combination matches the particular situation of a patient. This aesthetic is not concerned with the 'sublime', as in the beauty of art, but with a more unassuming form of beauty. Professional aesthetics are distinctly different from idiosyncratic interpretations of life aesthetics aimed at 'individual excellence', an Aristotelian twist. This would turn clinicians into artists rather than professionals, ignoring matters of the body, technology, knowledge and responsibility. Here it is self-effacing practicality, a nitty-gritty[20] professionalism that aims to fit to the situation of the individual, while the individual actively participates in this process. It resembles the functional aesthetics of tailors and carpenters rather than artists, where fit is a sine qua non for the beauty or elegance of the crafted object. A table or pair of trousers with one leg longer than the other(s) would be useless, rubbish, rather than a thing of beauty.[21] However, different from fixing a table or piece of clothing, care for chronic or terminal patients does not lead to a final product, because the situation of a patient keeps changing. The tinkering continues even after the patient is dead, for the relatives.[22]

Fitting individuals

Good care requires warmth and coldness, knowledge and empathy, but carers need to mix them in quantities that fit the particular and temporary situation of individual patients. This is in accordance with Sparrow & Sparrow's demands for individuality in the caring relation. How did the telecare system relate to individual situations? As a group, the observed patients underreported their suffering. This became very clear in the interviews: my informants did not like phoning doctors or nurses one little bit. They were afraid their call would come at an inconvenient time and be a bother to the nurse. This is a specificity of the patient group using the white box.

> Mr Johansen: It's a step you have to take. I am not really super sensitive to pain [*kleinzerig*], so when I went to the GP I had to introduce myself. I'd never seen the guy before. That was my medical history: there wasn't one. It's a big step for me, something has to be really wrong, I'd have to be sick as a dog before I'd call a doctor. But with the device, I keep them up to date, and if something is wrong, they call me. They get a red alert, and sometimes they call within five minutes. I imagine they read it when it suits them. I'm not bothering anyone, and my problem still gets attention.

Besides sharing the fear of causing disturbance, my informants saw themselves as realists – plain and sturdy people. They took pride in not running to the doctor for just any little pain. Rather than meeting the popular image of consumers actively demanding care, my informants spoke of themselves as reluctant to bother doctors. Patients in the other case studies for this book reported the same reluctance, but here they did explicitly link this to their own phlegmatic 'culture' – or nature.

> Mrs Dodijn: By nature I'm just normal, down-to-earth, Friesian, and if I
> have some little pain, I don't just run to the phone. It has to go on for a few
> days, and then I'll think: if it's not over by so and so, then I'll go.

One patient told a long, heartbreaking story about how her doctor *seemed*
to have *hinted* that she was a fraud, a hypochondriac reporting imaginary
complaints, because there was nothing to see on the scan. Although her
story made it clear that the doctor had not in fact said any of this, she was
still deeply hurt by what she saw as an attack on her own virtue, and her
care for herself and her doctor. The suggestion had broken the 'unspo-
ken agreement' between doctor and patient whereby she would not bother him and he would treat her complaints seriously when she finally
uttered them.

The telecare system and these particular patients – with their specific
virtues, concerns and reluctance to bother others – established an important fit. The system made a match between needs and ways of being. The
individuals shared particular characteristics, even if the device did not
address them, in a completely individualised way. There was a fit between device and human because the device interfered with the relevant
problems (e.g. patients who do not contact their doctors in time). Note
that the patients were not passive in making things fit. Patients could
also establish a fit when they refused to use the device, brought it back,
or took time and possibilities to adapt to its questions. This stopped mismatches turning into problems, as I discuss below. Fits are relational
products, as are warmth and coldness.

The notion of fitting

When 'making something fit' is a characteristic of caring relations between devices, carers and patients (or a group of patients and their
spouses), it becomes possible to understand giving medical information
as a way of caring, too. The notion of fitting makes it hard to label particular care content as either warm or cold regardless of the context it
would or would not fit in.

> Mrs Abenes: [The white box] asks some questions so often you get to know
> what they're all about. If you live through something, like being unable to
> sleep, you can see by the questions that insomnia is just part of the process.
> It comes back to you, it gets a name. That's really very nice.

The quote shows that the telecare system helps patients to name their
experiences and thus localise and give meaning to their feelings. Is your
insomnia a symptom of cancer? Or an effect of the chemotherapy? Or is
it just the flu, or, even worse, is there no explanation at all? The content
of the information is good, not because it is medical information, but

because it was relevant to Mrs Abenes and was given at the appropriate time.

> Mrs Veronica: I was in terrible pain after the first chemo. And I thought: 'If I have to go through this every time, oh that would be dreadful!' But that was the first time. I'm not someone to take pills easily. Usually I'd wait until I felt in pain and only then take my painkillers. But you have to keep ahead of the pain, not wait for it to come, because then you're too late. The device [white box] taught me this, so yes, it's really good. To make sure you don't get the pain you take the pills in advance.

The white box's advice released Mrs Veronica from the torment of her pain. That the fit is about sleep or pain, medical subjects or spiritual matters, is not a distinction of *a priori* interest to patients. They have concerns and complaints that may be both medical and social, and they are grateful for help with them. It would be unethical to hold Mrs Veronica by the hand and not help her take the painkillers in an effective way. The argument also holds for supposedly warm topics.

> Mr Frederiks: I'm an atheist. The question 'Do you find comfort in your philosophy of life?' has a religious perspective. If you are an atheist, it is impossible to find this kind of support in your viewpoints. To me, after death, it all stops. Others may think they go to heaven or the eternal hunting fields, or whatever they believe. But to me, it stops. I cannot find support in the fact that it stops, and they did not think about this when developing the telecare system.

Spirituality did not support this atheist. On the contrary, the question disheartened him for it did not take his minimalist philosophy of life into account. The mention of spiritual matters is not by definition comforting. Mr Frederiks does not consider it comforting that, after death, 'it all stops', even if others might find the thought of a heaven reassuring.

When 'fit' as a temporary result in the process of caring is a criterion for calling care good or not, the goodness of the intervention, be it medical or spiritual, is contingent on the relation. Neither warmth nor coldness has a pre-given meaning that is hidden in the essence or nature of the intervention. Both medical and spiritual interventions may be good, as long as they fit. Supposedly warm interventions may go cold when they discourage a patient. Empathy has a limit when a patient needs painkillers. Patients warmly welcome assumed cold interventions such as technical advice on how to use medication. Fitting is a relational activity, a way of interacting rather than an effect of machines. Users and devices have to continuously establish what may fit where.

Mrs Wilkens: You have to get used to it [the white box]. You have to get to know each other [laughs]. And you do that in a playful way. It's nice and easy!

Care that does not fit

People and devices establish fits interactively, but misfits as well. What misfits – i.e., failed attempts at good care – did I witness here? The patients complained about repetitive questions or unacceptable questions, for example on sexuality, which were regarded as an infringement of privacy. Some found it tiresome to read the long list of symptoms day after day if they did not have any, although it made some patients count their blessings. However, usually patients reported this as a minor nuisance. They could deal with it by skipping these questions or quickly running through them. They did not fit but did not disturb them either, and patients often kept the possibility open that they might become relevant later. The limited investment of time in dealing with misfits was a mollifying factor here.

The general protocol that made up the questions did not tune to individuals, but, paradoxically, this also helped the patients to deal with questions that did not fit their own situation. Apparently, the questions addressed other people.

Mrs Veronica: The white box asked about financial things. And that makes you think. I had some complications after my first chemo. Then you go out and buy things, but luckily we can afford it. And when I lie awake, I think about it: what do people do if they have to live off charity? They are just as sick as I am. It must be very hard for them when they have to buy things, like the expensive gel I bought to heal the blisters in my mouth. It made me think. And it made me sad. Some people can't do this so easily.

The inquiry about finances did not fit Mrs Veronica's situation, but she made it meaningful by relating it to hypothetical others around her. If it did not fit, it did no harm when the patients could situate the concern elsewhere, and they could even empathise with the implied others.

The most serious misfits were questions experienced as 'too confrontational', which only made a situation worse. A few people returned the white box in the first week of use.[23] They found it too strenuous (they were too ill) or too confronting, meaning that they did not want to think about questions of death and dying, possible symptoms or the impact of the disease on their lives because they experienced these matters as too intrusive and scary. The problems and refusals did not relate to placing care *at a distance*. The refusers and troubled patients felt the device was bringing care *too close* or made it excessive, comparable to the shopkeeper's complaint about his over-inquisitive clientele.[24]

The recurring example of a misfit initiated by the device was a set of questions on bedsores. The carers eventually modified these questions, but at the time of the study, the patients often discussed them. Mrs Jansen explained that they scared her. She was feeling well at the time and she was not thinking at all about becoming bedridden. The information on bedsores made her realise that having them was possible in her future too. She needed a lot of thinking to work out how to deal with this information.

> Mrs Jansen: You can look at it in another way. You can say: well, I might be in this situation, later. You have to think ahead, it *could* happen. But you don't always want to be confronted with it. But it is reality, it *could* be my reality. If you're prepared, you could deal with it better. You have to look on it like a maybe, not necessarily, but you *could* end up in this situation. Well, that's scary at first. Then you think: you should look at it another way.

It took Mrs Jansen lots of energy to make the bedsore information useful, or at least not harmful to her (it is a possibility, not a pre-determined fact, and if you do get them, you may as well be prepared). She had to do a lot of work to make a liveable fit that allowed her to relate to these questions. She described this as a *confrontation of worldviews*.

> Mrs Jansen: I refused it at first [when the white box was offered to her], because I was scared. Well, yes, I have my own views and they're optimistic. I told them I did not want to be put down in the dumps by the device. It would keep confronting you with questions you don't feel like answering. I don't want to change my view of life because of this device. I was scared it would press a pessimistic view onto me.

The difficulty with confrontational questions is to know *what* makes these questions confronting or unfitting. There was consensus on the misfit of questions about bedsores when one was not already bedridden. What surprised me was that it hardly ever concerned the idea of having an incurable disease. The patients who used the white box mostly dealt with this as a fact.

> Mrs Veronica: I'd looked at the questions [on the white box] with a friend, and she told me later that she found it all so terribly confronting. It said so clearly: you won't get better, asking questions like 'How do you see this, how do you deal with that, and are you sad about that?' She thought that was very confronting. But I said to her: 'Yes, but I *have* this disease. And I live with it.' So, to me, it's very different. I know I can't get better. They're doing lots to slow down the disease. But they can't stop it. So you know what the situation is. This is the way it is, I don't have a choice. I have to take it from there.

Users of the telecare system evidently could think about their incurable disease but, apparently, the refusers did not. The refusers feared that the telecare system would make their illness too central in their lives, unleashing their disease rather than taming it, blowing it up rather than reducing it to a manageable size. Indeed, patients engage in a relationship with a device that acts in their life. It is pivotal in that they may 'opt out' of such a relation when they feel it is impossible to deal with, excessive, or too hard to establish fits. When the relation establishes unneeded or untimely collisions rather than fits, care is harmful rather than good.

Modest aesthetics

'Warm' signified good care by its emphasis on ethical relations that respected patient subjectivity and acknowledged their feelings and thoughts. Cold care served as a critical term signifying an epistemological relation regarding patients' bodies as the object of knowledge that doctors should diagnose and treat. Doctors use objective parameters for this, such as lab tests and scientific knowledge, rather than patients' thoughts. The case of the white box demonstrated that putting both relations in opposition to each other does not help to analyse why patients experienced the telecare system as caring rather than as a cold technology. Even so, warmth alone does not fully describe what the practice of palliative care is about and why it works so well in Friesland. Elements of warm and cold, ethics and epistemology, subjectivity and objectivity are entangled. In practice, 'knowing patients' cannot be done without taking the experience of the patients into account. The patients need to sense and report 'when, how and where it hurts'. Respect comes from taking their treatment seriously and knowing when to apply empathy or when painkillers are the better option. When professionals do not look after bodies, empathy for pain is not ethical but cruel. When one professionally engages in caring, knowing the situation is also an ethical act, whereas ethically relating to patients is also a matter of using one's knowledge. In practice, the two do not exist separately.

So, both subjective and objective elements are part of a professional caring relation, but they cannot be neatly categorized into pre-established activities. Instead of separating and opposing warm and cold care, or ethics and knowledge, my analysis suggests a third metaphor to understand the goodness and badness of care, one that overcomes these fruitless oppositions: the metaphor of fitting. I analysed fitting as engaging in a practical and aesthetic relation between patient and carer or caring device. It is a *modest* aesthetics, lacking grandiosity or sublime beauty, acknowledging the limited possibilities for great results such as a permanent cure. It is also modest because the professional cannot control the process of caring; inevitably, the patients and their bodies play their part. It is a *professional* aesthetics, where professional stands for crafting and shaping fit, including the employment of clinical knowledge shared with other professionals that is needed to do what seems right. It is *contextual*, referring to the openness and sensitivity to the situation a patient is in at a particular moment. Clinicians need this sensitivity to evolving and unpredictable situations that are characteristic of the process of caring. And it is a *practical* aesthetics, where practical stands for the pragmatics of interventions; they need to be helpful to make the patient function as well as possible. *Aesthetics*, then, signify the beauty of a fit between relevant variables.

Like a good extension of a good clinician, the telecare system addressed a variety of relevant topics and their development over time (e.g. by repeating questions). It aimed for fits, trying to create them, avoiding and preventing misfits, and getting patients to help work on creating the fit. The telecare system would fail if it gave users no other option than to experience it as rude and unfeeling (as it did for refusers and with overly confrontational questions), if it made a wrong diagnosis or misinterpreted symptoms or when users would not engage in a relation with it out of indifference. As it happened, it did not reduce patients to their bodies or their minds but tended to both.

In an aesthetics of fitting, technology can be understood as caring – or not. Medical technologies are creative interventions that aim to transform the situation of a patient in order to improve it – even though, like Frankenstein's monster, their 'effects' are not in the hands of their designer and are not the sole product of the device alone. The role of users and their ideas of what care should look like is not passive and needs to be taken into account to understand 'effects'. People engage in real relations with technology. These relations may fail to improve situations or they may succeed, and both users and devices may initiate these failures. Essentially, it is no different from professional care by humans; but rather than just taking care's temperature, one might do better to look for the process of fitting interventions in the nitty-gritty order of the patients' lives (see also chapter 5).

Interestingly, the fitting here also relates to the mode of deliverance, that is, a device asking for response rather than a patient having to call a nurse. The patients did not experience their interaction with the device as impersonal or problematic but as supportive of their desire not to disturb their carers while helping them by staying in touch. Using the white box, patients acknowledged the subjectivity of their caregivers as well as their own.

So, should this be the end of metaphors of warm and cold? They cannot form a tenable opposition. Yet it may be too early to discard them. After all, as qualities of a relation between carer or caring device and patient, they did alert to the way in which affective relations between humans and technology may take shape. The metaphors discard a notion of technology, especially medical technology, as 'emotionally neutral' and merely functional. Affective relations with, say, cars, peak flow meters, insulin pens, computers, stamps and mobile phones, may prove to be an interesting topic for future research and an enrichment to comparable research in robotics and computers.[25]

3 The heart of the matter[1]

Good nursing at a distance

Goodness of fit

The metaphors of warm and cold point to the affective quality of relations between carers, devices and patients, where warm refers to loving,
good and well liked, and cold to unfeeling or neutral at best. Metaphors
of temperature drag along with them a set of influential yet – in care
practice – untenable oppositions, separating the objective from the subjective, the technical from the human, the ethical from the epistemological, and ultimately: the good from the bad. I have suggested a practical
aesthetics of fitting as a way to avoid this opposition.

The aesthetic verb 'fitting', however, may imply that fitting is about
authentic relations between individuals. Instead of the system world in-
vading the life world, everything would consist of intersubjective relations, including relations with devices. This is not a position I would
want to end up in. In this chapter I hope to show that fitting is not a
mere matching of people (or people and devices) but is situated in practices that include other devices, bodies, ideas about the world and – the
focus of this chapter – norms that define good care. For instance, in the
aesthetics of palliative care for people with incurable cancer, far more
professional care is deemed fitting than, say, in the care for people with
COPD or heart failure. The latter demands – and deems appropriate –
more activity and initiative from patients. Fitting care may aim for patient independence in some situations, whereas it would mean close professional monitoring in others.

In other words, fitting care is not merely dependent on the satisfaction
of the participants, it also takes shape by aligning care to the norms that
define good care. I understand norms of good care as *values* (say: good
relations, independence, cut-off points that define deviations) combined
with *directives* for what to do and who should do it (call or see a patient,
ask a patient to measure vital signs, prescribe medication). Both values
and directives are built into telecare devices[2] as well as activities of professionals and patients or in the ways they *enact*[3] good care. One needs to
ask whether the human participants see their acts as good or not, or *analyse their activities* as I do with the activity of devices, that is, within the
logic of the practice in which they are used. For example, devices assign
alerts in particular situations for the nurses to follow up. If nurses do not
follow up on an alert, this is not good according to the norm of the device. On the other hand, nurses may have good reasons for not following

up on the alarm. Care norms can be analysed, but following norms does not necessarily lead to good care. The result is debatable.

In this chapter I trace how *good nursing* norms enacted by the nurses and patients in this study changed when they started using telecare devices.[4] Particularly, I analyse what happened to the norms of good care that nurses were afraid might be threatened by the regular use of telecare devices. What new norms do nurses and telecare devices bring into being, and how do these relate to the ones already present?

The heart of good nursing

Nurses have particular concerns about telecare practices. The first is that telecare will upset their relationship with patients. The second concern is that telecare will stop nurses noticing signs of trouble in time since they are no longer seeing their patients at home or in the clinic. The worst consequence would be that patients suffer needlessly.

> Homecare nurse: As a nurse you have a kind of sixth sense. When you visit patients at home, you immediately sense if something is wrong. It's hard to put into words, but it's crucial for your work. If you use a webcam, you wouldn't, for instance, be able to smell the dirty dishes that have been lying about for a while. What would happen if you took that away? Wouldn't you destroy the heart of what it means to be a nurse? That's what I'm worried about.

The quote comes from notes I took at a European conference on telecare that was organised in the Netherlands in September 2007.[5] The conference was organised to discuss concerns and opportunities for telecare in the care for older people. The nurse's remark is typical of the kind of worry that nurses put forward in discussions on telecare. The professional fear is that telecare systems will make it harder for nurses to act competently and responsibly when looking after patients, because the nurse is not in the same space as the patient.[6] Although videoconferencing often gets a somewhat better press,[7] nurses often regard these and other forms of telecare such as sensors and monitoring devices with suspicion. The horror image is one of *cold negligence*: the patient is on telecare and gets worse without anybody noticing.[8] The final image is that the patient dies, isolated from the world, without relatives or carers, under the rational surveillance of electronic movement detectors, having felt the last supporting hand on their shoulder years ago. Telecare makes it impossible to use all the senses, let alone a sixth one, and the nurses worry about missing signs of trouble as well as losing human contact. This is a direct threat to 'the heart of good nursing'.[9]

Good nursing in practice

What did the introduction of telecare mean to nurses' relations with patients and the fear of neglect? I traced norms of good nursing in what I observed nurses and patients *doing* with the telecare devices (and the devices with them), in what nurses and patients *told* me about what they were doing and how they *value* this. I analysed material sourced from 12 specialist nurses observed or interviewed in depth. The informants came from five telecare projects based in three homecare organisations, seven hospital departments (cardiology & diabetes), a regional network of general practices and one homecare project for COPD patients.

Three devices were involved here, the first of which was a monitoring device for heart failure patients. Patients weigh themselves and measure their blood pressure daily. The devices transmit the measurement figures to a server where they are coded for deviations and made them available to nurses in a call centre. Patients can keep track of their own measurements on their TV. Call centre nurses monitor the daily figures; a sudden gain in weight may point to fluid retention that may, if neglected, be lethal to heart failure patients. Low blood pressure may point to medication problems. The call centre nurses follow up on deviations and discuss treatment options with the nurse in the hospital who is responsible for the patient.

The second device monitors patients by asking them questions daily. The 'white box' installed in the heart failure or COPD patient's home is a variation of the device analysed in the previous chapter. The white box, a health buddy, asks patients to observe their bodies for symptoms, as it did in the palliative care practice. In contrast to the palliative care practice, however, the white box also provides *education* and advice on good ways of living with heart failure or COPD. Specialist nurses in the hospital (in the case of heart failure and diabetes), in homecare (in the case of COPD) or assistants in general practices (in the case of diabetes) keep an eye on the answers that patients give and are warned by alarm signals if intervention is needed.

The third device is the webcam used by COPD patients associated with a homecare institute. Here, patients have weekly webcam contact with nurses. In addition, a touch screen gives patients access to a website offering entertainment and news on neighbourhood activities. A central Service Centre provides online bingo and other entertainment. The local homecare organisation is responsible for care. Email and internet is available to advanced users. One homecare organisation used both the webcam and the white box for COPD patients. I will mainly use examples from the first devices while using the webcam examples only to discuss the importance of meeting patients in the same space.

The importance of space

Chapter 2 discussed the nurses' most heated controversy in telecare technology: Would telecare come to replace contact with patients in the same space, and should this be a matter of concern? Why is actual contact in the same space so important for nurses? What would they lose if telecare removed or reduced actual contact? These questions are hard to answer. What exactly makes webcam contact so different from an actual visit? But even if many questions are still open, nurses are usually quite firm about one thing: without actually meeting patients, good nursing care is impossible.

> Specialist COPD nurse in homecare: I would never opt for 'just telecare' [in this case: using webcams]. As a professional nurse, I would quit the job if this was the case, if it was only care at a distance. I don't think you can deliver good care [when you are only working at a distance].

Why do carers say they need to see patients in real life? Obviously, hands-on care, as in washing and dressing patients, is impossible with care at a distance. It is also impossible to make a proper diagnosis. Professionals draw on a variety of information sources to make a diagnosis. For instance, besides talking to the patient, they may need to take blood or urine samples; besides observing the patient walking, they may need to examine their inner ear; they might need to use a stethoscope to investigate their lungs or might have to palpitate their chest; and even the sense of smell may be helpful to detect a disease or complication. Medical examinations require material visualization tools. There is also a consensus that some patients need home visits to 'sniff out' neglected households, which would signify trouble with the patient's condition. One specialist insists on personally meeting very ill patients:

> Cardiologist: Especially the very ill, you need to see them in person and get to know them. Individual circumstances make all the difference. 'Shortness of breath' may not mean much for one patient, but it may be a very severe symptom for the next. When you see patients face-to-face, you can see a lot, things that would escape you even if you have a webcam. The colour of the skin, the way someone walks towards you, a cold handshake or a pinched nose. Some things you have to really see and feel.

Webcam users always point to the visibility of the reactions of one's conversation partner as well as the greater chance of seeing and reading non-verbal signs (see Chapter 6). Seeing the other person draws the *visible body* into the conversation. This makes a webcam conversation more embodied than a telephone conversation, even if the bodies are not in the same space. Nurses using webcams still worry if this is good enough.

Homecare COPD nurse: Sometimes you have to feel people. Erm... it's different. A flat screen is only a flat screen, even if it is better than the phone. It's more intimate to actually meet. It's that *Fingerspitzengefühl* you get sitting beside someone in the same room. It's harder if you only see each other on the screen.

Fingerspitzengefühl (gut feeling) adds a sensory metaphor to understanding what is going on in a particular situation. In Dutch this is also referred to as the *pluis/niet pluis gevoel* (okay/not okay feeling), which senses the presence of trouble even if the source of the trouble has not yet been detected or made explicit. Nurses fear that these ways of sensing trouble will get lost if they only see patients through a webcam.

Another concern is the loss of non-verbal communication and how the physical position of bodies in space enacts ways of relating to a person.

Homecare COPD nurse: Sometimes you should stand or sit beside somebody. This is a real nursing task that doctors never, or rarely, perform. You put a hand on someone's shoulder, make physical contact, know what I mean?

The *position* of bodies is also part of the non-verbal conversation. Sitting in front of a screen, looking at the other's face, sets the stage for engaged conversations (see Chapter 6). Sitting beside somebody may signal empathy and support, even if there are no words or solutions.

So, reasons for actually meeting patients have to do with *required material* and the *embodiment* of certain forms of care. The material may be lab tests or handshakes but also the less explicit ways of discerning that something is not as it should be. An embodied presence is needed to 'sense' trouble and also to give the right kind of support, particularly when words are running out. Hence, nurses feel that a good relation between carer and cared for demands being in the same room.[10] Both the concern for noticing signs of trouble and patient relations are at stake here.

Division of labour

The importance of meeting patients in the same space is never questioned by the carers involved in telecare, but they may delegate *actual meetings* to particular professionals while others look after the telecare. This happened, for instance, when a call centre linked up with specialist heart failure teams in hospitals. The hospital nurses met patients in their offices, whereas the call centre nurses used the telecare device and the phone. The necessity of meeting the patient was uncontested. Or was it?

The call centre nurse told me how well she could do her job without seeing the patient. With some reshaping of new skills, she claimed she could work well with the telecare device and the phone. The new skills involved learning how to pose questions that would uncover the things she would have observed had she actually visited a patient. Although she stressed that the responsible heart failure nurse really should meet the patient, she felt confident *she* could do a proper nursing job even when telecare excluded the visual and the smelly bits.

> Call centre nurse: You can find out most things by asking the right questions. Like 'swollen ankles', you'd ask, for instance: 'Can you get your shoes on okay?' People tend to make things sound better than they really are. But in a social chat you'll soon notice if they are getting out to the shops or if they see their family.

The nurse directed the eyes of the patient to observe the relevant clinical signs for heart failure. But she did more than that. She invited the patient to chat about everyday life to focus the 'clinical eye' and interpret the signs for their relevance. In telling their stories, patients gave the nurse relevant information about their condition without being aware of it. Symptoms are retold in stories about everyday practices. Do patients get out to the shops, even if they say their ankles are okay?

Interestingly, being unable to see patients also revealed the *benefits* of not seeing patients. Here, telecare disconnects everyday life from useful information.

> Interviewer: What is it like sitting at the computer instead of visiting patients at home?
> Call centre nurse: That is a choice I've made. I want to do something for patients in my care, but I don't particularly want to *see* them. The good thing about not seeing patients is that somehow you start afresh. An image can distract. If you know what someone looks like, you can become prejudiced. There is lots of information you don't actually need, like if someone is smelly, or looks unkempt. We have a fixed list to go through: meds, allergies, history. It's a fresh image.

This nurse found a rationale where physical presence and visibility were not prerequisites for good nursing. In defining the information she needed to take care of people with heart failure, the call centre nurse excluded the way the patient dresses and smells as relevant signs. Good nursing meant concentrating on the physical condition and ignoring distracting impressions.

This is a big change from the idea of the sixth sense needed to spot *any* kind of trouble, which is also a way of saying that different problems *relate*. Symptoms may not be so easily distinguishable from other problems.

Homecare COPD nurse: We want to know how the patients feel, emotionally, and also physically. 'How did you get up this morning? How is your medication?' Often people have their own questions. Sometimes it's just hot air, so to speak, just chatter about household stuff. And that is the nursing side of it: you should be able to do that, too; you listen between the lines. You jump on the signs you read between the lines. It could be that so-and-so's sister-in-law is really ill. You talk about it, because it has an impact on how he is. You look at the total picture of the patient, not just the COPD, the whole patient really. How they're doing in life.

The call centre nurse did not spot ill sisters-in-law or 'whole patients'. She spotted weight and blood pressure deviations. Therefore, this particular telecare device *specialised* the nurse's observations, while at the same time the daily measurements *intensified* them. The nurse established the link with daily life practices only if shifts in vital signs gave reason for phone calls.

So, carers strongly defended the necessity of actually meeting patients, even if they did not do this themselves. Telecare practices where nurses did not see patients, however, also challenged this 'rock bottom of clinical knowledge'. Nurses thought about forms of care that did not need meetings with patients in the same space. At the same time, the monitoring system changed *what* problems were relevant to watch out for. It reduced the chance of spotting relevant signs in any situation, but it increased the frequency of monitoring specific symptoms. Only when the monitored figures started deviating did the nurse retrieve older and broader norms to interpret the deviations.

Keeping up old standards: correcting telecare

Another general objection to putting telecare to work is that devices presumably standardise care at the expense of individually tailored care (see Chapter 2). This is not valid for webcam telecare but may apply to other devices. The next example is from a hospital ward for heart failure patients. There was a clash between a particular norm of good 'care as usual' and the norms inscribed in the educational device, a variant of the white box. The educational device tried to implement a general norm for the right way of living with heart failure. The white box asked patients about their weight, physical activity, salt intake, fruit rations, cholesterol level, medication, and so on. The protocol defined norms that fit *all* heart failure patients: be careful with salt, and exercise is good. The alarm labels signalled any deviation from these general lifestyle rules; this was the clinical relevance that the device's script supplied.

This general recipe for good patient care turned out to challenge norms of flexibility, individually tailored care and clinical relevance in 'care as usual'. Here, nurses attempted to tune their care to the individual's situation. They found that giving information on medication to patients who did not take it, as sometimes happened with the white box, was confusing and wrong. They insisted that signs and symptoms were only relevant if they fitted the patient's specific situation.

The conflict between general advice and individual situations became clear when Maartje Schermer and I[11] interviewed 83-year-old Mrs Smit, who did not see the point of taking physical exercise even though the white box told her that she should. When the white box asked if she had exercised, she answered 'no'. This sent an alert to the nurses' office, which the nurses followed up. When they called, Mrs Smit explained that at her age she did not feel like exercising. The nurses accepted this.

> Heart failure nurse: You keep an eye on things, and if everything is stable, I don't complain. Some people choose not to follow the advice. One woman just says: 'It's all right by me, this box and all these questions, but I won't always do what it says. I'll only eat salt-free three days a week. I can't do more than that.' If someone manages, one way or another, and they're in good condition, you shouldn't make things stricter than necessary.

Happily for the patients, the nurses held on to their norms of good nursing and stuck to the personalised treatment. But sadly for the nurses, this implied a more complicated relation with the telecare device. The device kept sending alerts to the nurses, even when 'deals' had been made with particular patients. Technicians could not change this for individuals, as the nurses learned from them, which probably had to do with the difficulty of making exceptions to a general protocol. In this case, the nurses worked around the norms imposed by the device and kept up their preferred norms of good nursing.

Yet doing this came at a price for the *nurses*. It meant that if they knew the patients and accepted their particular ways of living, they had to ignore the alerts that warned of this 'agreed deviation' of the protocol. The alerts could not be – and were not – used at face value, but nurses needed to connect them to the patient's background. The nurses had to make the fit between general norms and individual situations. The nurses tackled this problem by reading *all* the answers of all the 66 patients in their telecare project and by establishing their own criteria for judging them, phoning up patients when they were in doubt. This was an option because the nurses had a limited number of patients involved in the pilot project. It would be different if more patients used the device, or if nurses were more pressed for time. If nurses do not know their patients, you can expect many false alarms.

So there was a clash between norms. There were the general lifestyle rules versus tailor-made care; there was efficiency in informing many patients versus tailored information. Extra work by the nurses provided the answer to saving the perceived best norm: tailor-made care. Telecare put an extra burden on nurses to correct the problems the device introduced in order to ensure that telecare fit their idea of good care. Hence, relations between nurses and patients remained good and even became closer (see below). Rather than missing out on trouble, the devices identified a *surplus* of problems. It was up to the nurses to distinguish between them.

Telecare as an improvement: changing norms

In the first examples, telecare was seen as an *addition* that cautiously challenged meetings in the clinic or at home. Nurses also saw telecare devices as *complicating* factors when tailor-made care was the ideal and devices brought in general protocols. The devices also created new problems, such as the many false alarms or incomprehensible signals. There were, however, also arguments for seeing telecare as an *improvement* to care as usual. When this happened, consultations at home or in the clinic ceased to be the gold standard of care. It substantially changed ways of thinking about good care.

From health status to process

How can telecare do better than care in the same space? At a meeting with call centre staff, the project coordinator and the call centre nurse monitoring heart failure symptoms discussed what care for heart failure patients is all about.

> Project coordinator: 'Time and attention are very important to patients. What happens with heart failure? You go to hospital, time is limited, and if they solve one problem one day, the next problem will pop up the next day. Patients don't take it all in at once, they forget to ask about the things they wanted to ask.'
> Call centre nurse: 'It's always hard for these patients to accept that they are ill. It takes them a lot of time.'
> Project coordinator: 'Quality of life comes first in our project, it's most important. Quality is in the daily grind. And in education and practical advice on looking after yourself' [she adds quickly].

The call centre staff told me that the monitoring system lets them tend better to changeable trouble in the 'daily grind' of living with disease. Daily monitoring, they claim, means they can tend to the *process* of illness better than encounters in the clinic once every three months would. The situation of the patient changes over time, they encounter new problems, and so it helps to check the patient frequently. And unlike visits to the clinic, the patient is free to call in whenever he or she wants to discuss worries. Even if frequent phone calls established such relations with only some patients, this is the general idea. Frequent monitoring – and calling – makes a high frequency of patient contact possible *and* attractive. In the same vein, the object of care and concern changes from health status to process, adapting the question from 'How have you been feeling these past three months?' to 'What's up today?'. Instead of a patient history, they address the patient's here and now. This changes how nurses get to *know* their patients.

The daily delivery of signs from patients and the availability of frequent contact made nurses keen spotters of trouble when it arose, particularly in the project using the white box with heart failure patients. Patients informed nurses every day about an abundance of topics.

> Heart failure nurse in hospital: You get to see patients earlier, yes, you're right on top of it! People don't always call when that's the advice on the white box. You'd be lucky if they come into hospital when they're having a bad time. But if they don't call, they'd end up in a hospital bed. You can't always prevent that, but now you're right on top of it all.

Nurses can be 'on top of it all' because they call their patients if they discover that something is out of order. Patients rarely called the nurse in this practice, even when the telecare device urged them to call. This reluctance to call also came up with the Friesian oncology patients and the homecare COPD patients. The device corrected this by sending information that would warn the nurse when something was wrong. When it happened, the nurse could respond quickly and call the patient. Nurses knew something was wrong at an early stage, even if the patients had not called. So the frequency of the telecare communications emphasised good care as interventions in the day-to-day process of tending to illness. In contrast, consultations every three months now seemed badly timed.

Interestingly, the homecare nurses using webcams reported another effect of more frequent contact. They did not find that weekly webcam chats added further information to the answers generated by the white box, nor did webcam chats reach the depth of the three-monthly personal encounters in the clinic.

> Homecare COPD nurse: I noticed the [webcam] contacts became superficial. When patients come in every three months, you talk for half an hour, using the protocol for all the questions you want to go into. You discuss smoking, for instance. If you meet on the webcam, you don't discuss smoking every week. It's rather: how are you and what's happened this week?

In the cases of monitoring symptoms or responses to standardised questions, stable patients do not demand attention, even if the white box provided a seemingly endless list of topics. In webcam conversations, they do. The monitoring practices may thus hide the symbolic meaning of 'daily checks'; they would be particularly useful for patients going through many ups and downs. Exhaustive questionnaires add a few extra patients. Patients, however, often felt the daily monitoring was a comfort, even when their illness was stable. Telecare intensified the role of the professional.

From self-care to professional monitoring

For patients, daily connection to the nurses induced feelings of safety in any telecare setting, regardless of whether they were actually experiencing problems. They thought that the nurse would be the best judge if something was wrong.

> Mr Danick: If they took it [the monitoring system] away from me, it would be like taking my phone. Some of your security would disappear. Of course, you know a lot, because you have lots of experience with your heart and with your body. But this is the next step, so to speak. It feels safer. The thought that there are people out there checking on you puts you at rest.

The patients saw their relations with the nurse improve through the frequent contact. The nurses also experienced closeness but related this to their phone calls with patients.

> Heart failure nurse [talking about the white box]: What we notice, especially in the beginning, is that patients give answers that need a response. So the phone contact with new connections is really intense. One way or another, you get more familiar with these people, even on the phone. You get good contact. They start trusting you, 'Hey, they'll call me if there is something.' To them, that's a revelation, really.

The safe feeling that patients experienced came from the regular checks and their experience of the nurses calling them if something was out of the ordinary. The patients' satisfaction with this may be related to the fact that many people with a chronic disease are *scared*. In the words of Henriëtte Langstrup: 'for patients, telecare practices seem to treat *fear* rather than symptoms.'[12] This may well be true, although fear often relates closely to symptoms. Being rid of fear may also mean a reduction of symptoms such as breathlessness.

> Mrs Jansen, homecare COPD patient: If you get scared or insecure, you get out of breath. Because fear gives you cramp. Then I'm glad when I'm out of breath that I can talk to them [the nurses] about it. I have a son, but you don't want to bother him all the time. It gives you a breather [*lucht op*], takes away the tension that builds up when you're sitting here alone, when you get breathless. I can't quite explain it but...

The nurses felt that their more permanent presence in patients' lives would have a therapeutic effect in the long run. The telecare nurse served as a reminder that some tasks were still open, particularly for patients needing to change their lifestyle.

> Homecare COPD nurse: You see people becoming more aware. They sometimes say: 'I don't want to be confronted by my illness all the time.' But even so, they need to change their habits. It matters if you keep an eye on that from a distance. It gives the patient the feeling, 'someone is looking over my shoulder, I'll have to do something'. For instance, if you saw [COPD] patients in the consultation room, you'd talk to them about quitting smoking. You'd discuss the consequences of smoking. Whenever they visited you, they'd say: 'I really want to quit smoking, but not quite yet.' In the end they come and say: 'I want to do it.' So when you're watching them constantly from the background, the problem stays up front.

Even if frequent webcam contacts were superficial, they still served the purpose of keeping patients alert.

The increased frequency of contact meant a big change in nurse-patient relations. The nurse no longer just reacted to the patient's questions or problems discovered in the quarterly clinical encounters. In the telecare projects, the nurse exerted more professional control, foregoing any ideals of leaving the initiative to ask for help with the patient or making patients responsible for their own care. This meant a shift from a reactive, reticent form of nursing to the prevention of crises.[13] Nurses taking responsibility for prevention gave patients peace of mind. The patients trusted that nurses would keep them out of harm's way or would act if they could not avoid harm.

Ironically, professionally guided telecare fits well with the nurses' fear of negligence and their urge to spot trouble. The nurses may have found their mechanical sixth sense in the very practice they feared would take it away – that is, in using telecare devices. Especially practices that allowed them to address different problems daily gave nurses the sense of being on top of things. The patients were happy with the increased professional care and the good relations they had with their nurses. To them, sending out information was a way of having the nurses check them daily, and the nurses' follow-up was a welcome addition that initially surprised them but in the end made them feel safe.

> Mr Welvoorden: When I got that box, I thought: what a load of rubbish! You get a whole load of questions, yes, no, one, two, three, all answers are good. So I gave the wrong answer, on purpose. And half an hour later, the phone rang. That's how I tested it, to see if it worked. Then I did it again a few weeks later, because maybe they only check new patients. But again, the phone rang! So they really do something with it.

Both patients and nurses saw telecare involving daily input from the patients as a fitting improvement. It signalled trouble quickly so that nurses could intervene quickly to avoid crises. Older values that were previously deemed fitting, such as patient responsibility and caution with medical intervention, tacitly disappeared.

New tasks, new goals

So far, the new norms developed in new telecare practices have dealt with treatment or guidance for patients, and this was what the task designers intended for the telecare devices. In the following example, this link with patient care was broken. The potential of telecare unleashed the nurses' creativity and let them invent new tasks and goals for their device. It started when the heart failure nurses realised that as an educational device, the white box was teaching them new things about their patients, different from what they would have learned in actual meetings.

> Heart failure nurse: We were stunned by the answers people gave. It made us think: 'What is this? Doesn't he know *that*?!' All of a sudden you get an enormous amount of information from a patient, stuff you wouldn't get in the half hour of face-to-face contact. So the white box is a great way of getting to know a patient's missing bits.

The 'bits' missed in the quarterly consultations took specific shape: they were facts about the disease that patients did not know. It could often be very many facts, so new topics became a matter of concern. The white box identified the problems in the variety of questions it posed throughout the months. Problems related to mood and sexuality worried the nurses. The patient might mention these topics in a personal consultation, but the problems could remain invisible if patients did not report them out of embarrassment or other reasons.

> Heart failure nurse: The answers are far less 'socially desirable'. On the one hand, they feel safe, because they know somebody is there. But on the other hand, it doesn't bother them to fill out a questionnaire. I'm sure that if you asked some people about their weekly salt intake, they'd say: 'Oh I never take salt.' But when the question is put on the white box, they'll answer: 'I take salt three, four days a week.' See? They're far more honest. That's surprising, really. Rarely does someone tell the white box that they stick to a completely salt-free diet.

Seeing the answers from *many* patients, corrected for social desirability, made the nurses wonder: what do we know about mood and sex-related problems for people with heart failure? How can we find out if these problems affect many patients and maybe add something to the care we deliver in order to help change these problems?

> Nurse: If 80 out of 100 patients give the wrong answer to a certain question, you should look at yourself – not at the patient, but at how you explain things to them. It's a way of checking to see if you're getting stuff across the right way, asking yourself "How can we do that better?"

White box usage shifted away from facilitating treatment and became instead a tool that heart failure nurses used to study the care they gave. Rather than acting like hands-on (or phones-on) clinicians, the nurses became *researchers* of their own practices. The object of their research was different from the object of clinical practice: it was not the case of the individual patient but the characteristics of the *group* of heart failure patients that the nurses were researching.

To fit this new goal of research, nurses had to make singular observations gained through the telecare device meaningful in new ways. Taken out of context, it was not always clear what the answers meant. Was a patient just reporting a blue day? Or did the blue day point to a depression that needed treatment? Taken out of context, it was not clear how reliable one observation was. The nurses wanted to collect statistics from the group of patients so that they could aggregate the scores for all patients and find out, for example, how often depressed feelings were reported and if certain problems were typical for this patient group.

Sadly, at this point, the device that had first unleashed the nurses' enthusiasm now tamed their excitement. The software could not handle creating statistics for the whole group. The only graphs possible summarised data for individuals only. So the nurses figured out different ways of getting the information needed – for example, by sending out paper questionnaires to assess depression. Although the device may have unleashed the idea, the nurses did the actual work to achieve what they now thought was important for good patient care.

The shift to quantitative data collection and interpretation meant a shift towards embedding a form of local epidemiological research in clinical practice. To the nurses, this was a valuable option because it fit their norms of good nursing. Again, telecare helped to uncover *more* problems that patients might have. Moreover, the telecare device corrected a problem with face-to-face contact: patients may be too shy or too reluctant to disappoint the nurse to talk about problems that are easy to confess to a white box. This appealed greatly to nurses who were worried they would oversee any problems suffered by patients.

Persistent values, shifting norms

Telecare did not brashly overrule the norms important to good nursing. On the contrary, telecare turned out to strengthen some of these norms. The nurses in the study were firm about the importance they attached to contact in the same space and to maintaining good relations with their patients. Even if some nurses delegated personal contact to others and pointed to the problems of these actual meetings, their importance was unchallenged. Contrary to what they had expected, the nurses succeeded in using telecare systems to create even *closer* relations, through frequent contact and by responding to the signals sent. They maintained their link with individual patients despite the sometimes heavy demand for extra work put on them by the telecare systems.

Telecare did not seem to endanger problem-spotting. In the practice of the white box, the number of possible problems to spot increased. However, in the monitoring practice the problem content changed as well as the frequency. The nurse's expertise in 'reading' symptoms in daily situations at home remained important. Mouldy dishes seen firsthand could point to a degree of breathlessness that might not let the patient get to the kitchen. Creative nurses, however, could make these observations on the phone. Patients might not report swollen ankles, but they might be tempted into telling the nurse what they had been up to lately. However, before these 'broad views' of *any* sign of trouble came into play, the type of problems nurses thought fit to signal changed in the monitoring practices. The monitoring system brought about a reduction and specialisation in problem types, but it also intensified monitoring.

Thus, there is both continuity (broad values persist) and change; the way to enact good relations, the problems to target and how to do this changes. More frequent monitoring brought the possibly daily shifting process of illness to the foreground. Hence, nurses felt they could respond far more readily to problems than they could in hospital visits every three months. They explored other possibilities for identifying problems by imagining using telecare for research. Here again, the problems changed, this time from those of individual patients to the problems of the group of patients. Changing objectives and problem definitions also brought a change in values. Responsibility shifted to the nurse, away from the patient, and the value shifted to prevention and away from self-help and cautious medical intervention. Consequently, patients felt safe (rather than responsible) and well looked after by their nurses. To them, telecaring nurses took the place of their own vigilance in preventing crises.

Contestable norms

These findings do not suggest that nurses need to worry about a *reduction* in the quality of relations with patients or in their ability to spot problems. Instead, telecare could lead to *over*-involvement and problems targeted *too frequently*. There is a fit between the nurses' use of telecare and the values that nurses take as central in care, even though other values entered their practices as well. The nurses could only establish this fit, however, when they could link 'data' to individuals, particularly when it concerned the use of the white box. When nurses were unfamiliar with patients using the white box, they would have many more 'false positives' to follow up.

The feeling of security the patients experienced was an intriguing finding that deserves more reflection. These feelings may not always be realistic. Patients still have chronic and potentially fatal diseases, and telecare does not take that away. One woman became very cross because she had a heart attack, despite sending in her vital sign measurements twice a day. When fear is an important problem and a recurring theme for COPD and heart failure patients, this suggests that it deserves attention. The best way of dealing with this is a discussion I would like to open up. It is also unclear how feelings of security may relate to the responsibilities that professionals cannot take on. Patients may be discouraged from looking after themselves. This is a huge leap from the promise that telecare would promote self-management of their care. The patients in the practices I studied became passive rather than active, although some webcam practices succeeded in setting up 'communities of care' between patients (see Chapter 4).

The analysis shows that fitting caring relations is more complicated than merely assessing if the 'carer' and 'cared for' are both happy with their relations, devices and activities. Fitting does not only take place in relations between patients, devices and carers but between different norms in care as well. These norms do not always go together easily. Increased professional control is at odds with norms of self-management by patients. Relations in which the patients feel safe and the nurses feel on top are excellent for both parties. Yet one may nevertheless argue about the desirability of these norms. This may become even clearer when one compares monitoring practices with alternative practices and different norms of living with disease. The next chapter compares the ways in which two devices support very different ways of living with chronic disease.

PART II

Knowledge and promises

4 Caring for the self?

Enacting problems, solutions and forms of knowledge

Shaping problems

In this chapter, I look at the ways devices and their users solve particular problems together and how, by enacting remedies together, *they shape what these problems are*. Problems are defined by particular knowledge (e.g. physiology) within which some variables fit (e.g. overactive angiotensin-converting enzymes) and others do not (e.g. trouble getting to the shops). The second problem would be relevant in the clinic and at home, but doctors may or may not translate it in physiological terms. Hence, the *terms* describing problems and the *practices* in which they are enacted matter to the form a certain problem takes.[1]

There are various ways to describe the patients' problems. Devices contain various forms of knowledge, and patients and carers enact yet other versions in their activities. Using different forms of knowledge means that different facts are relevant to understanding what is wrong with patients, as in the physiology and housekeeping problems described above. You can learn about these forms of knowledge by asking participants in care practices to tell you how they understand and deal with patients' troubles or by studying the context in which devices are used and facts are enacted.

My analysis in Chapter 3 described norms as containing values as well as directives. Knowledge in care practices contains *facts* as well as directives. The directives are, for example, on how to *obtain* knowledge and on how to *solve* the identified problems. For example, the overactive enzymes suggest treatment with drugs (ACE inhibitors, to be precise), whereas the problem of getting to the shops may demand the purchase of a mobility scooter. The directives connect and enact facts and values simultaneously. Another example: patients and nurses enact the daily process of illness (fact) by frequent measurement (directive) to facilitate quick intervention (value).

This chapter zooms in on the situation of *patients*, analysing the various problems, solutions and ways of living with chronic disease that are enacted in two care practices by patients using two different types of telecare devices.[2] I demonstrate that both practices contain different kinds of knowledge about the problem and about how the patient cares for this problem. The chapter outlines the kinds of self-care that patients engage in. 'Self' and 'care' have no fixed meaning here but will be shown to differ in and between telecare practices.[3] The place of experience is, for instance, very different in both practices, and so is the way the tele-care solution relates to the forms of self-care that patients already use. I show that patients never care for themselves alone but rather together with devices, professionals, family, friends and fellow patients, in various configurations.

In this demonstration, I analyse the situation of two chronically ill women, Mrs Jansen and Mrs Jaspersen. Both are fictional compilations of real patients, put together to include the elements needed for the presentation of this analysis. The quotes are real but stem from various real patients. Each situation sketched here features another telecare device that co-shapes knowledge on the possible problem and invites patients to engage in particular forms of self-care. The telecare device is not the only form of care in the lives of the patients. Telecare co-exists with other ways of defining and solving problems.

Mrs Jansen and the heart monitor

Mrs Jansen suffers from heart failure. This means that her heart is failing to pump blood properly around her body, placing Mrs Jansen in acute danger of retaining fluid. If she retains too much fluid, it may fill her lungs, and this would mean the end of Mrs Jansen. Obviously, she and her doctors must find ways to prevent this from happening. Mrs Jansen has to stick to a strict diet that regulates her salt and fluid intake, and she does not know which she finds harder to live with – less salt or less fluids. She cannot drink more than 1.5 litres a day and she has to avoid eating salt. To keep an eye on her condition, Mrs Jansen is 'on the monitor', as she puts it. Every day she weighs herself on the special scales that she has in her house, and after that she measures her blood pressure. The monitor transmits the daily measurements to the hospital, where the heart failure nurse checks them. Should anything be out of order, the nurse will call Mrs Jansen to discuss what she needs to do. A sudden weight gain might signify fluid retention; low blood pressure might point to trouble with medication.

Mrs Jansen is encouraged to call the nurse herself if she feels something is wrong or if she notices that her weight or blood pressure measures go beyond set thresholds. But this, she says, she will not do. She does not want to bother the nurse. 'In most instances, it passes,' she explains to me. She says she can spot fluid retention: it makes her ankles swell. When in doubt, she used to step on her own scales to check her weight, although she does not do this anymore now that she has the telecare scales. If she sees she is retaining fluid, she lies down for an hour or so and it goes away. And if it does not, she might take an extra half or a whole diuretic pill. 'The doctor said I could do that!' she assures me, as if I were accusing her of trespassing on the doctor's territory. She also takes ACE inhibitors, but her doctor does not let her tinker with those.

I ask her why she needs the monitor if she seems to have things under control anyway. Mrs Jansen shrugs and says it is nice to have it. She feels safe having the nurse keeping an eye on things. 'Of course you know a lot, because you have lots of experience with your heart and with your body. But this feels safer. The idea that there are people out there checking on you puts your mind at rest. They know a lot more about heart failure than I do.'

Mrs Jaspersen and the webcam

Mrs Jaspersen suffers from COPD (chronic obstructive pulmonary disease), a progressive lung disease. It used to be called emphysema, signifying that the lungs lose their elasticity and become prone to inflammations that may lead to immediate hospitalisation. The disease makes breathing difficult, and Mrs Jaspersen gets out of breath quickly. After walking a hundred metres, she has to sit down to recover. Shopping was a truly athletic endeavour for her, until she was no longer able to do it. Then Mrs Jaspersen became desperate. After consulting her GP, they admitted her to a rehabilitation clinic where she learned to live with severe COPD. Her 'life, body and soul', as she put it, were turned inside out to find potential improvements, from breathing and walking techniques to pacing her energy and panic control, and from medication to daily routines and exercise. Upon her discharge from the clinic, a computer with a webcam was delivered to Mrs Jaspersen's home. She can use the computer to surf the internet, check email, and use the webcam to talk to others on a closed network of fellow patients from the clinic. In the three months following her discharge, she had weekly webcam meetings with her carer from the rehabilitation clinic.

When does Mrs Jaspersen use the webcam to talk to other patients? 'When I'm not feeling well or looking for distraction. Then you think a lot of things: would my illness be coming back, is the hospital waiting for me again? Then I talk to my friend to find out how *she* feels and what may be wrong.'

Mrs Jaspersen continues: 'She [the webcam friend] told me some crazy things. She said that when she gets out of breath, she puts two chairs beside her own, one to the left, one to the right, and then she puts her arms on the back of the chairs.' Mrs Jaspersen looks at me slyly, as if daring me to challenge her. Having convinced herself that I am interested, she adds: 'You know what? I tried it and it really helps me too!' Mrs Jaspersen points out how she has pre-set the chairs inconspicuously around her dining table so that she can quickly take up this pose by moving only one chair. Dragging furniture around is not easy when you are out of breath! The arrangement had to be subtle; there is no other option when one wants the house to look spick and span at all times. Mrs Jaspersen also points to a bag filled with boxes of medication. If she feels a crisis coming up, she has to take her own antibiotics and prednisone to avoid hospitalisation, involving a drip with a mixture of corticos-teroids and antibiotics. The clinic encourages her to take advantage of this ability to self-medicate. Mrs Jaspersen can recall the exact date of her last ride in the ambulance for emergency admission to hospital; it was more than two years ago now.

Enacted trouble: objective symptoms versus subjective experience

Two women, two devices, two chronic diseases and several possibilities for support. Both women use different forms of knowledge brought in by various means and persons, aimed at different problems. Mrs Jansen has her measurements, the diet, the educated and experienced nurse, the bed rest, diuretics and ACE inhibitors. Mrs Jaspersen has the web-cam, her fellow patients, the chairs, the carer in the clinic, the bag of medication, internet and email. Each of these implies ways of under-standing what is wrong and suggests possible things to do in a particular case. The telecare device is but one of various possibilities. Let's analyse these care practices more closely to see how different problems are en-acted.

Monitored disease

Let's take Mrs Jansen's monitoring device. By weighing and measuring herself, Mrs Jansen produces figures. If blood pressure or weight values deviate from their individually defined standards, that is defined as a problem. This applies if either value crosses the threshold set by the cardiologist. The computer protocol will detect it and send an alert to the nurse, who will then call Mrs Jansen.

> Mrs Jansen: Well, they [the nurses from the call centre] are really nice and friendly people, honestly. It's, well, just... See, my weight is usually between 62 and 63 kilos and one day it went up to 63.1, well, this one little ounce may be gone the next day, but me, I got called straight away. I think this is over the top.

Although one ounce may not seem like much to Mrs Jansen, according to the logic of the device, it does cross the threshold value. This is what thresholds are for: to signal when they are crossed, whether that is by a little or a lot. The only way out of this would be to change the threshold levels.

Organising problem identification like this separates subjective com-plaints from objective measurements. When you measure objective parameters in a patient's body, the nurse does not have to wait for Mrs Jansen to report complaints. The purpose of measurement is to warn of trouble, and this creates the difference between what devices do and what people experience in their own bodies. Value deviations may be ignored or go unnoticed, or complaints may be reported without the figures running wild. In the case of monitoring heart failure patients, this difference is even more important because, as the telecare project leader told me, these patients tend to underreport complaints. They actually feel, or pretend to feel, better than is warranted by the objective measurements. Close monitoring makes it possible to intervene when it is *necessary*, meaning when the numbers signal *real* trouble. The monitoring device, or so the project leader argued, enables nurses to see patients faster, before things get out of hand.

The device does not target the problem of people who feel *worse* than they really are. These patients either go to their doctor or suffer in silence. Sticking to the logic of objective disease means that the doctor may reassure them by pointing out that their values are okay or the doctor might tackle the less vital problems. If they stayed at home they might *feel* miserable, but nothing would *actually* be wrong with them – that is to say, nothing directly related to their failing heart. They may be suffering but they do not need life-saving intervention. Their bodies are fine; a glance at the figures proves this. So, with the nurse watching over the daily measurements, the monitoring device favours objective measurements more than subjective complaints. This makes sense when complaints are unreliable, meaning they do not point to a relevant physical reality. The monitoring device thus corrects unreliable subjective experiences of the disease.

What is made to matter here is the condition of a body that may be objectified but is hard to know subjectively. Mrs Jansen's comment that the nurse 'knows best' is understandable. The nurse has the knowledge to distinguish relevant symptoms and knows how to interpret the signs that no longer belong to the patient's subjective realm of experience. But what is this subjective experience? Mrs Jansen tells me that she *knows* when her body is retaining fluid. She may not feel it but she can certainly *see* her swollen ankles. And she is perfectly capable of interpreting the measurements herself, even if she does not do this. Thus the measuring device does not merely *objectify disease*, it also *shifts responsibility* for spotting trouble from the patient to the nurse. As such, it competes with Mrs Jansen's other practices in self-care and troubleshooting. For instance, Mrs Jansen has the discretion to adapt her dosage of diuretics and handles the ways to shape her diet and deal with reduced fluid intake. Crises remain, however, the responsibility of the nurse.

The nurse 'manning' the monitoring device in the call centre encourages patients to call and share whatever worries they have. However, patients like Mrs Jansen hardly ever call. According to the nurse, people start confiding in her only after she has spoken to them on the phone a few times. When this happens, the call centre nurse develops quite intimate relations with the patients.

Nurse: People can always call, whenever they like [during office hours].
Interviewer: Do they call you when they get a new grandchild?
Nurse: [laughs] Yes, we get to know those things. One time a patient called to tell me exactly that.

The team is looking for ways to phone people more often to develop this closer contact and was preparing information videos at the time of the study. At that point, however, the set-up facilitated objective symptom monitoring better than any discussion of complaints and personal worries.

Webcam worries

Now let's turn to the care practice of Mrs Jaspersen. What kinds of problems are enacted using webcams in follow-up care? Typically, the webcam does not script the *content* of problems in any structured manner, as was the case with Mrs Jansen's monitoring device. Patients can communicate anything discussable by webcam, from vital signs to leisure time, and from breathlessness to domestic affairs. The various communication partners connected to the webcam network multiply this 'anything'. Apart from the carer, there are the fellow patients. A clear directive from the webcam is, however, that patients address problems by making *webcam contact*, to explore and pinpoint what these problems are *interactively*.

Let's see what problems were mentioned during the interviews and the observations in the clinic. On the webcam with her caregiver, Mrs Jaspersen discusses her treatment plan and any troubles she is having in adapting her daily life to what she has learned in the clinic. The carer is happy with virtual meetings on the webcam because patients like Mrs Jaspersen may feel embarrassed to 'confess' explicitly when they are not doing so well. They are not unreliable reporters without a clue of their true condition, but they feel embarrassed about asking for more help when they have already had so much. The consequences of stating explicitly that something is wrong can be far-reaching: every patient fears hospitalisation.

Mrs Jaspersen: My social worker, she knew me so well, and the [webcam] vision was so clear, she could spot right away if I was lying to her.
Interviewer: Lying?
Mrs Jaspersen: Well, in a manner of speaking. If I just sat there, looking at her, she'd say: 'I can see by your eyes that you are not doing well.' So, that's the advantage of a good [webcam] system.

The webcam helps to overcome the barriers in reporting trouble, not by objectifying symptoms but by extending the trust and intimacy of the caring relations established in the clinic. The carers can *see* when things are not well; they know the patients and they know what they look like when they are doing well and when they are not. They use intimate knowledge of *this* particular patient to observe if there is any trouble. For instance, Mrs Jaspersen always dresses well, so it would be immediately obvious that something was wrong if she showed up for her webcam session in a dressing gown. Mrs Jaspersen told me that her carer knows her so well that she always gets tailor-made advice, even more than from her carers at home. The webcam uses the familiarity of the webcam partners to identify problems (see also Chapter 6), and support therapy (see Chapter 3).

Mrs Jansen also uses the webcam to talk to fellow patients when she is not feeling well, she said, but also 'just for a chat'. A couple of fellow patients from the rehabilitation clinic have become her close friends. It is not hard to take the initiative to contact them, especially when there is trouble. The others can identify with her problems and they are very happy to support each other, all having been in the same position themselves.

When Mrs Jaspersen is worried for whatever reason, she can call a fellow patient. The existence of a relationship prior to the one developed over the webcam turns out to be a condition for benefiting from the visual potential of the webcam. Without this relationship, visibility did not add much relevant information, and patients even saw it as too intrusive for talks with 'strangers' (see Chapter 6). It is the same for the carer: familiarity with the other is a condition for the webcam to function like this.

But fellow patients share more than friendship. They share knowledge. They know what it means to live with COPD and to have to fight for breath. Mrs Jaspersen could call on her friend, the expert, to help her find out what might be wrong with her. Together they might compare their shared phenomenology as COPD sufferers.

Gunvar, Jane and Rose, three COPD patients, are chatting in the rehabilitation clinic

Gunvar doesn't often use perfume even though she loves wearing it. 'If I put some on, it makes me gasp for breath. But,' Gunvar adds, 'then I just open the window, and my breathlessness is gone. I don't worry about it.'

Jane mentions a perfume by name, adding, 'It's the only brand that doesn't take my breath away.'

They talk about Rose, who told the others that she gets out of breath from cooking smells. Jane does not believe her. 'I think she is exaggerating.' Gunvar defends Rose. 'It's different for everyone.' But none of them can bear aerosols.

Here, the problem is not one ailment in a single defective body but rather the sharing of the experience of living under the various conditions related to COPD. Air pollution, panic attacks and weather conditions all influence breathlessness, and all need solutions other than medication. Everyone mentions they feel depressed at times, and web-cam support often successfully cheers people up. The patients recognise the problems and think about them collectively. Illness connects them, not primarily in a disease category but by a set of physical, emotional and practical variables that they share and can develop knowledge about (more on this in the next chapter).

Fellow patients could articulate more problems together. For example, they discussed the *invisibility* of their symptoms to ignorant others, which made them feel misunderstood and misjudged.

> Mrs Jaspersen: What I find really very hard about this disease is that you can't tell from the outside that someone is ill. Sometimes I'm better than at other times. People just don't have a clue what it means. When I told my neighbour about my emphysema [the term formerly used for COPD] she just said: 'Oh, my grandson has eczema, too.' Really, people have no idea.

Apart from being misjudged by others, there was also the trouble they *themselves* had in seeing that they were ill or accepting their illness, as they and their carers would put it. All patients had experienced the trap of 'getting it wrong' and overburdening their bodies on a good day. Accepting that one has a particular disease, however, implies far more than mental acts of 'facing the facts'. It implies new ways of behaving, observing the variations in one's condition and capabilities, learning how to negotiate the changes and reacting with what one deems to be important to do despite the difficulties. The patients must get to know themselves anew and learn what they can do. They may learn this in the rehabilitation clinic: to acquire a new sense of what to do when old routines have let them down. The active re-interpretation of physical symptoms and the retraining of their bodies involves a tough learning process. The process is not merely a psychological matter; it is something the *body* has to learn as well.

> Mrs Jaspersen: You see, once you get out of breath, you think everything is going to happen, you think this or that, you think you're going to die. But no, you should try to synchronise your breathing with your mind. Then you'll be okay again.

Simply breathing and getting out of breath sends the wrong signs, explains Mrs Jaspersen. It leads to panic and an acute fear of dying. What she had to learn was to 'synchronise her breathing with her mind' – that is to say, to breathe not on automatic pilot as always but in a new way that depended on self-reflection and practice before it became routine. In this case it would be to 'talk back' to her body ('You are not dying') and teach it a new response ('Sit down, don't panic, try to breath normally, check if you need to take a pill'). It is to re-educate and resocialise the lived body. Together, the befriended COPD patients made these problems visible by articulating them as shared problems. They supported each other in building a new understanding of themselves as 'bodies with invisible disease' and 'bodies having trouble understanding breathing difficulties' and live accordingly.

These examples show a knowledge of daily life with COPD that is shared, actively developed and used by people living with the condition. The exchange and development of this knowledge are embedded in both friendly and professional relations. This is a big contrast to Mrs Jansen's practice. Mrs Jansen had to deal with the tensions arising from unreliable subjective experiences and symptoms objectified by the monitoring care practice, and she was responsible for finding out other things by herself. In her own practice, however, Mrs Jaspersen's experience forms the starting point and points to a shared reality of living with disease and access to shared knowledge that comes with this. The knowledge is not about reporting symptoms to caregivers (both patient groups seem to be bad at this) but about living with them. Familiar others are helpful here. They may confirm trouble or explain it by comparing things to their own situation or ways of experiencing the world, or to how they know their friends behave. Mrs Jaspersen's group actively produces knowledge that is relevant to their present condition.

Here, experience is not suspect or in need of correction; patients can shape it productively, share and sharpen it with fellow patients. It is knowledge about 'living with a condition on a day-to-day basis'. It is different from professional knowledge because it stems from embodied experience and shared skills (see Chapter 5 for more on this).

Articulating problems

So, in these two care practices, different problems emerged as relevant, requiring different knowledge and a different place for patients' experiences. Obtaining this knowledge required different activities by different actors (patients, professionals, devices, medication). These problems were not 'already there' but were actively shaped to create a fit between the devices, the role of the carers and the distribution of responsibilities. Monitoring vital signs helped establish an objective disease in the body, whereas the webcam encouraged interactive problem definitions using the patients' experiences and observations. Vital signs connected with professional interpretation. Interactively defining problems needed knowledgeable friends with phenomenological insight into their responses and appearance.

Although I have not yet analysed the 'care' invoked, clearly 'self-care' is never just about the 'self' or one single body. *Who* cares for *what* problem is not set in stone – it shifts. Devices took their part, professionals took or were appointed particular positions, and fellow patients were or were not consulted. There were combinations of at times contradictory strategies and knowledge. There were bodies carrying objective diseases, and bodies with shared concerns. In each genre of presenting facts about problems, the 'self' was a different entity with different problems and different parts to play.[4] The patients' role emerged in the material setting and in their use of available strategies, which created the distribution of responsibility among patients, professionals and devices. Telecare devices helped to unleash or tame some versions of disease rather than others.

Responding to problems

What patients are supposed to *do* about their problems differed in the practices of Mrs Jansen and Mrs Jaspersen. It depends on the way problems are identified. As became clear, the different settings shaped 'the self' and 'disease' differently, but what did 'care' come to mean?

Measurements

Let's go back to Mrs Jansen and her monitoring device. Patients like Mrs Jansen are invited to put on and inflate the cuff to measure their blood pressure and step on the scales to weigh themselves. They have to do this every day to provide the figures for the nurses. It must be a daily routine because of the nature of *measurement*. A single measure on its own is meaningless and unreliable. Patients may be unreliable reporters of their own disease; they also have to correct for the unreliability of the monitoring devices – or the amateur patient's use of them – by frequent, routine measurement.

> Mrs Jansen: It's part of what you do, your life. How shall I put it. I get up in the morning, go to the loo and step on the scales. And then we have breakfast. And after that I take my blood pressure and everything. It's all part of the routine. And once all of that is done, I can get on with my day.

Patients need to produce measurements for extended periods. Their disease is chronic; the figures may shift at any time. The measurements that patients produce with their devices should ultimately lead to warnings of possible trouble. And this is where the nurse comes in. The *nurse* has to make sense of the figures and come up with a solution. The division of labour in the monitoring practice seems to be that patients are responsible for producing the figures via the telecare system, while nurses are responsible for encouraging them to do so, interpreting the figures and coming up with a remedy if needed. The participants tacitly agreed upon this – Mrs Jansen by her passive waiting for a call and the nurse by her active calling.

The patients were glad to leave it to the nurse to contact them. Mrs Jansen said: 'I'm happy to be looked after by someone who knows more about my condition than I do.' Even if Mrs Jansen *knows* something is wrong, the nurse and patient will use the monitoring device to establish professional control at home anyway. It makes Mrs Jansen feel safe and allows the nurse to spot trouble as soon as it appears. She does not wait for patients to call her but intervenes when it is timely. So, in this care practice, patients are more actively involved in their own care than they were before the telecare device arrived: their action is in the realm of 'taking daily measurements' and following the instructions of the nurse. When it comes to *interpreting* symptoms and treatment decisions, the monitoring system intensifies professional care rather than delegating it to the patient. Patients appreciate this: they feel safe and taken care of because the nurses monitor them.

The responsible nurse caring for symptoms contrasts with Mrs Jansen's need to maintain a salt-free diet, mind her fluid intake and manage her diuretic medication. She had to figure these things out for herself and had to decide if and when she needed professional help. At the time of the study, the call centre staff was working on an information campaign. They sent out informative videos – for instance on prescribed diets – for patients to watch at home. However, the videos did not go down well. The videos were made in America and did not fit Dutch practices – or attitudes – in a straightforward match.[5] The nurses intended to send patients good salt-free recipes, using spices instead of salt for seasoning. They planned to spread ideas on how to keep fluid intake low on hot days, for example, by sucking on frozen pieces of pineapple. They did not address diuretic use, since not all patients took them independently.

The life of Mrs Jansen shows three configurations of self-care. First, there is the monitoring practice where Mrs Jansen is, above all, a patient suffering a disease needing specialist care. Self-care thus takes on the form of 'doing the legwork' for the nurses. Second, there were the emergency diuretics or resting in case of fluid retention. The clinicians left it to Mrs Jansen's discretion to take a pill or take a rest, although the nurse may make suggestions too. But Mrs Jansen never calls her. These self-care options target the same symptoms as telecare devices do (fluid retention), but their logic is quite different, particularly because the patient herself is responsible. This responsibility exists although medication is considered a 'medical' solution, and lying down is not. Third, there was the daily inconvenience of coping with the diet and reduced fluids. Again, Mrs Jansen was responsible for this, although plans for support in this area were in preparation at the time of the study. The nurse *may* address these matters should the figures start to deviate. However, patients dealt with them as they thought fit, and doing so allowed them to balance the importance of diet against their other assignments in life.[6]

How do these self-care configurations relate? In the practices studied, they do not relate at all other than the fact that Mrs Jansen had somehow to live with them all together. The introduction of telecare did not relate to whatever the patients had been doing before; most patients were already watching their weight or signs of fluid retention, if not as systematically as in the monitoring practice and not in digital form. More systematic monitoring and control by the nurse now replaced homemade pencil-and-paper monitoring or accompanied ankle observations as well as a great degree of discretion in matters of using diuretic medication or dieting. Ways of caring for oneself followed quite different logics.

Mutual support

What type of self-care did Mrs Jaspersen's practice of using the webcam put forward? Clearly, videoconferencing helped bring about care that interactively shaped problems as well as solutions. If something was wrong, the webcam invited patients to get help and share their experiences. This served to articulate what the problem was and address it at the same time. What remedies did the patients come up with? The first remedy was social diversion. Taking your mind off the hardship of living with chronic progressive disease may be a good thing every once in a while. Webcams allow you social contact without having to leave the house.

> Mrs Jaspersen: One time, I was a bit down in the dumps, so to speak. So I went to the computer and what happens? Suddenly, another patient calls me up. Well, you go sit at that thing [the computer] and you don't feel well, and so on. Then this fellow patient calls you and you start chatting. And [swears], when you're done you're a completely different person! I noticed that a few times. [...] Or playing some game or another on your computer distracts you, so your breathing gets more relaxed. Because you're not paying attention.

The computer and the webcam promote another form of self-care too: patients 'broaden their horizon' by engaging in meaningful activities rather than just focusing on their illness. Although it takes great effort and much training to get elderly patients comfortably using a computer, this effort allows new problems to emerge and provide new ways to solve them. The result here was that supposedly technophobic elderly patients such as Mrs Jaspersen started using email and surfing the internet. Mrs Jaspersen stopped just focusing on what was wrong with her and looked for positive things to do in her life, by 'bringing the world into her home' and by caring for her friends.

Now wait a minute. Down in the dumps? Diversion? Loneliness? Broadening horizons and finding meaningful things to do? Could these be medical issues? What the problem is as well as ways of solving it may indeed be articulated along different lines than what is often understood

as 'medical'. The webcam shapes and addresses a fluid mixture of physical, social, emotional and practical problems and solutions, and stages
events in the midst of many routines of 'getting through the day'. These
are all ways of making life bearable. The self-help in this practice aimed
to do just that: help patients live their daily life.

The webcam also allowed patients to address the difficulties related to
symptoms and to share and refine the solutions. Take the three-chair
solution Mrs Jaspersen learned from her friend: rest your arms on two
adjacent chairs to ease your breathing. Mrs Jaspersen *refined* this techni-
que by integrating the required set-up of chairs into her normal furniture arrangement. This meant she could position herself quickly without
having to shuffle around or move the dining room chairs every time the
need to breathe better got in the way of the demands of having a tidy
house. This remedy relieves symptoms, and yet the doctor may not
know of it. It connects different goals of equal importance (alleviating
breathlessness versus keeping a tidy house). It is an invention created
by patients living with breathlessness.

Interestingly, it is not *despite* but *because* of the shared problem of living with COPD that Mrs Jaspersen developed an extensive support network. She receives care and support, and she herself is a *carer and sup-
porter* as well, lending her expertise to others. She can be active and take
the initiative to look for help. As a collective, the patients share the care
for each other and engage in reciprocal or *'together-management'* of their
lives.[7]

Mrs Jaspersen's self-care practices were comparable with the discretion that Mrs Jansen was given over her diuretic medication (I analyse
this more closely in Chapter 5). And Mrs Jaspersen encountered practices of objectifying disease in the body as well. She visits a pulmonary
specialist every year to have her lung capacity measured. As an intervention in daily life, Mrs Jaspersen is less than happy about this (more analysis of this point too in the next chapter). Overall, using the webcam was
not at odds with how Mrs Jaspersen was accustomed to care for herself.
The webcam extended her network and gave her alternatives for consulting professionals.

Enacting problems, engaging in self-care

Different enactments of problems and self-care imply a different appreciation of patients' experiences and know-how. The more their experience is questioned, the less often patients are addressed as responsible
partners in their own care, as 'self-' or rather 'together-managers'. The
professionals and telecare device took care of monitoring objective
symptoms. The patients had little access to the parameters monitored
and lacked the knowledge to find solutions when these were out of line.
Mrs Jansen observed her body retaining fluid but did not do this by

monitoring her personal measurements – instead, she observed her ankles. The monitoring practice did not relate well to Mrs Jansen's other self-care practices and these were sometimes inconsistent, especially regarding who was responsible for what; they merely co-existed next to one another.

The more socially or interactively enacted problems facilitated by the webcam helped turn experience into *knowledge*. This process brought other potential carers into the picture such as fellow patients, people who shared Mrs Jaspersen's specific interests and ways of living with disease. Framing issues as problems of daily life made professional responsibility and expertise only one (much valued) source of solutions. It actively engaged patients in identifying their worries and finding the best way to deal with them.[8]

Self-care gained different meanings. It turns out that it is misleading to think in terms of one patient (one self) caring for the self. The work is always distributed among patients, professionals, devices and others. The self of the patient may do more or less work, take more or less responsibility, or be more or less creative. This self is, however, never by itself. Devices, professional carers, objects, regimes and other people shape it together.[9] The term 'self-care' or 'self-management' glosses over these interdependencies. Indeed, together-management would be a better term, granted that the devices are included in the 'together'.[10]

But what about the *care* aspect of self-care? As shown, there is no single rationality or epistemology underlying the practices of living with a disease. There are many rationalities, including professional surveillance, responsibility for medication, or for bringing the world into one's home. Patients tinkered with various logics of care[11] for themselves, piecing them together using particular strategies for particular problems. You could say the telecare devices tinkered with the patients too, since the devices permitted several ways of using them and had their restraints as well. Webcams made it easier to contact others in case of trouble. The monitoring system with the nurse 'at the other end' led to the nurse rather than the patient taking action.

Different telecare systems supported different ways of living with chronic disease. There is no single way of doing this that follows from the 'nature of a disease'. The *type* of disease does not determine care; COPD patients may objectify their condition, for instance by blowing into peak flow meters or by having their lung functions measured. Heart failure patients, in turn, could also use webcams. This would not exempt them from the task of keeping an eye on their weight and fluid intake, but it would make other knowledge and activities important as well and enable another kind of life with chronic disease. It makes the question of what device to use, and a fitting logic to live by, important for potential users to ask.

Fitting logics

The previous three chapters have shown the processes of fitting devices and people, fitting norms of good care as well as fitting forms of knowledge. This chapter makes clear that fitting responds to and establishes various logics of care. There are also relations *between* logics. These logics could co-exist in the practices of an individual patient – either hampering or supporting one another. But there are also clear differences between the practices of Mrs Jansen and Mrs Jaspersen living with monitoring devices or webcams respectively. Different logics of care become apparent: values (quick detection of problems versus mutual support), facts (problem identification by vital sign deviation versus discussing personal experience) and directives may or may not become routines (measurements versus mutual support). In the next chapter I look in more detail at the knowledge that patients need for fitting – and switching between – various logics in their daily lives.

5 Knowing patients

On practical knowledge for living with chronic disease

The knowledge of patients

In the previous chapter, the examples of Mrs Jansen and Mrs Jaspersen and their respective telecare devices showed how they used norms and knowledge from different logics they had to somehow fit together. To the facts, values and directives derived from devices and professionals, both women added their own experiences. By using the webcam, Mrs Jaspersen could develop yet a different kind of knowledge by sharing her concerns about living with COPD with her fellow patients. In this chapter, I look at how people with severe COPD use knowledge in their daily life practices to deal with their disease and the things they want to do in life. What kind of knowledge is this? How does it relate to professional knowledge? How can telecare devices such as the webcam support the development and use of this knowledge?

Studying the knowledge of patients is, however, easier said than done. There is much opacity on what this knowledge could be about and how to study it. The main pitfalls seem to be either completely *separating* the knowledge of patients from medical science and technology or making them *the same*. A way out of these difficulties is to *ignore* the knowledge of patients and professionals for the greater good of 'empowering' patients. Obviously, this does not help much to put the knowledge of patients on the research agenda, even if it does greatly influence ways of thinking about patients and what they can and should do. Before analysing the practices of people with COPD, I will briefly consider these problems, in order to avoid them and prepare the tools for the analysis.

Knowing patients?

The question of what the knowledge of patients is must be placed in the context of the emancipation of patients. The days are long gone when doctors and others saw patients as passive and ignorant lay people dependent on and sometimes abused by medical/research practices.[1] Modern patients have gained influence in medical practices and in the production of medical knowledge. Health care policies, laws and guidelines have been developed and implemented to protect and make use of the new position of patients.[2] What happened to the knowledge of patients in this process?

Difference

There have been attempts to study the knowledge of patients as 'knowledge by experience'. Patients obtain this knowledge by living with a chronic disease or disability. Much confusion surrounds the term. There is the danger of romanticising experiential knowledge by defining it as *essentially different* from medical knowledge.[3] A romantic notion of knowledge by experience risks trivialising this knowledge; it is not 'real' knowledge but the 'exotic' lay wisdom of patients.[4] It may be meaningful to them but may be completely wrong according to professional medical standards. There is no reason to trust its claim to truth.[5] Defining experiential knowledge as different from medical knowledge is also problematic in a high-tech medical world. In the life of chronic patients such as the ones described in this book, medical knowledge is everywhere, in the form of devices, medication, lifestyle rules and so on. This knowledge does not always fit but is difficult to ignore as part of the patients' experience and expertise.[6]

Sameness

The term experiential knowledge often pops up in situations where medical experts do not recognise diseases[7], in the case of 'orphan diseases' lacking medical research[8] or where patients find medical knowledge and interventions unhelpful.[9] Experiential knowledge is then the only knowledge available, and these patients organise themselves in their struggle to gain medical recognition for their disease and to promote medical research to understand and treat it. Here, experiential knowledge runs the risk of switching from being essentially *different* from scientific medical knowledge into becoming generally *the same* as scientific medical knowledge. The patients become what Epstein calls 'lay experts' – well-informed patients who discuss science on an equal basis with scientists.[10] The difference between what patients and their organisations know and what medical science may extend and confirm is roughly that medical scientists have access to laboratories and scientific methods, whereas patients develop their knowledge 'in the wild'.[11] Although the tension between patient experience and 'evidence' is far from resolved, patients do engage in the production of medical knowledge or guidelines.[12] The *production* of knowledge has changed in the process, but not the *object* of this knowledge nor the *methodology* to develop it.

The call for scientific medical knowledge is widespread, and the idea that this knowledge is the same as the knowledge that patients might use and help to develop is very common. Another example is the policy of self-management. The self-managing patients as described in the UK policy on the 'expert patient',[13] for instance, and in the discourse on the modern 'informed patient'[14] get hold of medical technologies to support themselves. The most cherished technology is the internet, which provides all the medical information anyone might need and gives access to a variety of aids, portals and discussion platforms. The idea is that equipping patients with the right technology – and this certainly includes telecare – will help patients to manage themselves, their bodies and their diseases. Patients get to know as much about their disease as their doctor does, if not more. After all, they have only one specialisation to keep up with.

To equate the knowledge of patients with state-of-the-art scientific medical knowledge, as the above examples do, obscures the translations that patients (and clinicians!) need to make in order to make scientific knowledge useful. It is nothing new to state that statistics, for instance on groups of patients, are not directly applicable to individuals.[15, 16] The patient in the doctor's surgery may have complicating co-morbidities that patients in the study did not have. Patients may gamble on the idea that they are the exception to the rule ('My granny smoked and she lived to be 95'), or find that treatments do not work in their individual case. To make scientific knowledge useful to them, something has to happen to it. Patients need to translate this knowledge and tinker with it to fit the particular situation at hand.

Indifference

Equating scientific knowledge with patients' knowledge makes the latter invisible as an object of study in its own right. This is also the case in discourses on dominance in doctor-patient relations that assume that differences in *power* should be the focus of attention rather than knowledge. The idea is that societies should enhance the power of patients, not by learning about their rationality but by taking their emotions, choices and preferences seriously. This discourse frames the patient as a *consumer*, a character that shows up in several places.[17] This type of patient, for instance, plays a political role in the Dutch health care market as the 'third party' counterbalancing the power of health care providers and insurance companies.[18] Consumer-patients may do this by negotiating with decision makers, by refusing to accept care they do not want, and by declining to pay too much for the care they *do* want. For consumers it is not important what they *know*, but what they *want*.

The consumer-patient also makes an appearance in theories about evidence-based medicine (EBM). To reconcile medical rationality with patient preferences, EBM frames the patient as given the choice between two equally effective treatments. Irrationality does not get free rein, because doctors are supposed to have only evidence-based treatments on offer.[19] In the *juridical* sense, however, the consumer-patient is free to prefer and choose anything, even if their choices do not fit with medical rationality or will lead to the certain death of the patient.[20] The patient is, legally speaking, autonomous.[21]

Tools for the case study: scientific versus practical knowledge

The ideas of 'exotic' knowledge, expert patients and active consumers did not help to put the knowledge of patients onto the research agenda. When *exotic*, the knowledge of patients would not be analysed as knowledge but as perspectives or beliefs. An analysis of patients' knowledge would be *irrelevant* when it is taken to be the *same* as scientific medical knowledge, or *superfluous* when the power to choose is deemed more important than sharing knowledge. In this chapter I will use a contrast between *practical* and *scientific* knowledge to study the knowledge of people with COPD. This contrast allows for distinctions between medical knowledge created by scientists, clinical knowledge from professionals, and practical knowledge from patients, without losing sight of their complex intertwinements.

The idea of contrasting practical and scientific knowledge is based on the work of Georges Canguilhem.[22, 23] On the one hand, there is what Canguilhem calls *the laboratory*, meaning the formalised or scientific knowledge that presents transportable and comparable facts. This knowledge comes in different versions or logics that separate enzymes from anatomy and genes from epidemiology.[24] *The clinic*, on the other hand, signifies the knowledge that doctors need to treat individual patients. Clinical and scientific knowledge generally differ in their aims. Scientific practices aim to generate knowledge about the way bodies behave in particular conditions. Clinical knowledge does not aim to accumulate knowledge but to improve the daily life of individual patients. To this end, clinical knowledge feeds from numerous sources such as the scientific literature, medical tests, patients reporting trouble, and so on.

Another difference between scientific and clinical knowledge is the way in which they are legitimized. Scientific knowledge comes with procedures for creating this knowledge that the scientific community has agreed on. Clinical knowledge derives its authority and reliability from the experience of the clinician and builds on many observations of patients' reactions to treatment and advice, as well as the ongoing process of observing, intervening and evaluating *this* particular case.[25, 26] Does the patient improve? If not, what could be the next step? Clinical knowledge is about tinkering and adjusting rather than finding evidence.[27] It is about improving rather than proving.[28]

Practical knowledge for clinicians and patients

If clinical knowledge is the practical knowledge of professionals, it is possible to extend Canguillhem's reasoning to think about the practical knowledge of patients.[29, 30] There are, however, also differences between the two. The clinician aims to treat or support individual patients, whereas individual patients aim to live with their disease in a good way.

The clinician knows how to *instruct* patients; the latter need to be good at *putting instructions into practice*. This is a difference between *explicit* and *tacit* knowledge. Polanyi showed that tacit knowledge is not necessarily explicit, or it has ceased being explicit.[31] It is embodied. The bicycle rider relies on many tacit routines that would take much effort to articulate. This does not mean that one cannot make tacit knowledge explicit, although philosophers argue about the extent to which this is possible.

Another difference is that patients move through several practices beyond the clinic, constantly finding new situations to deal with. The patient may *talk* about these situations to the clinician but primarily has to *live* them. Dick Willems gives a useful example when he set the stage for a GP, Bob, and a patient, Susan. Susan suffers from asthma and Bob gives her an inhaler to help reduce her breathlessness.[32] As a GP, Bob is perfectly able to *explain* to Susan how to use the inhaler. Susan, however, is the expert when it comes to the embodied skill of *using* the device and in using it inconspicuously and conveniently in everyday life. She not only needs know-how to do this, she must also interpret new situations to know if she needs to use the inhaler or not. Explicit 'knowing about know-how' may be shared between patients and professionals. Actual embodied knowledge is, however, specific to those living it. It is not exotic but rather highly dependent on the specific situations in which they find themselves.[33]

Practical knowledge of people with COPD

These concepts enable me to differentiate between forms of knowledge without having to deny their interdependencies. I will now turn to my case study of practical knowledge of people suffering from chronic obstructive pulmonary disease (COPD) to see what they are worth 'in the wild'.[34] The people with COPD struggle to shape their lives and their disease, helped by the people around them and the technology they use. My analysis draws on fieldwork in the rehabilitation clinic for COPD and asthma that Mrs Jaspersen from the previous chapter visited as well. I conducted follow-up interviews with patients who were using webcams to stay in touch with each other and the clinic. I also conducted fieldwork in the clinic to study how patients and carers use webcams and how volunteers trained the patients to use computers. When I questioned how this device fit into the daily life of the patients and how they used it to transport what they had learned in the clinic back home, I learned a great deal about the strategies and obstacles of living with COPD on a daily basis and gathered many examples of their practical knowledge.

I distinguish three levels of practical knowledge in the practices of COPD patients (see Table 1). The first is explicit knowledge. Theorists sometimes call this propositional or declarative knowledge, which is formed from statements of fact or propositions about the world (for example: oil does not dissolve in water). The second level of knowledge is based on know-how or skills and is sometimes called procedural knowledge. This knowledge is embodied or embedded in routines and provides techniques and methods. Skills may be enacted or expressed and may be applied in particular situations. An example is skill in using inhalers or in baking apple pies.

The third level emerged from the study of the practice of patients with COPD. I have dubbed this category *know-now* to indicate the activity of knowing in a particular situation. Patients use *know-now* when they *interpret* new situations to establish what the problem is and how they should act. *Know-now* is about asking open questions – What is the matter here? What should I do about it? – instead of giving answers or applying skills. For example: 'How should I interpret that red spot on my face? Does it need treatment? Is it a sign of the measles; is it eczema, acne or something else altogether?' Patients also need *know-now* to coordinate knowledge from different sources and logics.

Table 2 Levels of practical knowledge

Propositional knowledge[35]	Know-how	Know-now
Statements or propositions	Skills	Semiotic problems
Descriptive, declarative	Directives & routines	Open questions: what is ...?
Matters of fact	Methods & procedures	Tools
General	Specific to (familiar) task	Specific to (new) situation
Explicit facts	Tacit embodied knowledge[36]	Sensitising concepts
Valid in different situations	Experience	Improvisation
Detached from person's body	Body as source of knowledge	Body as instrument
Result	Method	Observation
Knowing that	Knowing how	Knowing here & now
White box[37]	Monitoring device[38]	Webcam

Introducing 'know-now'

COPD patients clearly displayed both tacit and explicit pragmatics in their practical knowledge. They needed directives and suggestions for 'what to do' to improve their daily life or keep it stable. Interviewing patients who had left the clinic, I asked what they had learned in the clinic. Only occasionally did they treat me to stories on the chemical composition of drugs or the physiology of lungs extracting oxygen from air. Mostly, their answers were about *practical arrangements* that allowed them to interpret, respond to and deal with the breathlessness they faced in their daily lives.

The term 'know-how' refers to a set of tacitly and automatically applied skills. If you look at the practices of COPD patients, skills are indeed important, but *many* are involved and their application (which skill to use when) was not straightforward. What seemed more urgent were resources that allowed people to *improvise* in new situations, to 'know-now'. This means they looked for ways to understand and act in *this* particular situation. Here is an example.

> Mrs Smit: I learned [in the clinic] that you should focus on getting to know your limitations, and also that you have to make these limitations explicit. So when you are doing sports and you should stop: how can you let others know? How can you tell you've reached a limit, how do you deal with that? A lot of work in the clinic aims at that: that you need to recognise your limits and learn what to do with them.

This practical knowledge gives Mrs Smit pointers to things she should be aware of: her limits. A related element is the proposition that one should 'respect' these limits. However, the patients must assess the actual meaning of 'respect' and 'limits' in concrete situations. A limit is temporary and situated. It gains meaning only when it is encountered in a specific situation; it is know-*now*. 'Limits' functions as a sensitising concept, not a definitive one.[39]

After Mrs Smit has sensed and identified the nature of a particular problem (or limit), she has to figure out what to do. This requires an assessment of the context and those in it as well as a strategy to deal with it. Should she explain her disease to people? Merely wave to signal that she will wait behind? In Lucy Suchman's terms, situated action is called for rather than plan implementation.[40] Mrs Smit must improvise, using what she knows about the situation and about different ways of dealing with problems.

In the quote, questions form the tools for assessing the situation: Is this a limit? What kind of limit is it? How can I deal with it? These questions are *specific* and *open* at the same time. They are tools or methods for understanding a situation and finding out what to do in it. It is the active verb of *knowing* rather than the noun of *knowledge*. Every set of activities needs to be sensed and thought through in terms of expended energy and new arrangements to be made in order to best live them. The practical rationality needed here demands solutions to new puzzles and calculations with ever-changing sets of variables.

> Mrs Matthijsen: You have to think more when you do things – that's what I learned. You sort things out: if I do this, I can't do that. Tonight, for instance, I have a meeting. And I said: Let's make it at my place so I don't have to go up and down four flights of stairs. Before, I'd just go and work out how on earth I'd get up the stairs again when I got back.

Mrs Matthijsen uses the expression 'sorting out' a problem. In this example, the stairs formed the problem. On other days, it may be something else. She needs a kind of knowledge that allows her to assess and find ways to deal with different circumstances.

Know-now points to the process of understanding. In the rehabilitation clinic, but especially in the webcam practice, patients could be seen to develop *know-now together*, by assessing someone's situation together. They do this, for instance, when they are trying to understand the reasons for their breathlessness. Does it relate to cold weather, air pressure, pollution, lung inflammation or something else? The webcam patients form an active community of *know-now* producers to identify and solve emerging problems. Here is an example of how the webcam helped the COPD patients practise *know-now* together.

> Mr van Leeuwen: The contact with fellow patients is really nice. There's always a night when you wake up short of breath, things are not working out, and then you think: Is this me, is it my illness, or what? If you can talk to another patient and he or she feels just as bad, then you think: Well, I'm not the only one suffering today. Then it turns out that there is a storm depression coming or weather like that. That has the same effect on you as going up a mountain: less air pressure. If your breathing is bad and there's less oxygen in the air, you notice it right off, definitely. And then you see: Well, it's not just me.

A law of physics – less air pressure equals less oxygen, which makes breathing more strenuous – a proposition is included in this knowledge. But *know-now* is not aimed at establishing this proposition, it is used to help diagnose a particular situation and find ways to react to it. Mr van Leeuwen and his webcam companion are trying to learn what their bodies are doing at a particular time. They are not sure *why* they are getting out of breath. But being out of breath in thundery weather is something you can *sense*, it is a reaction to be expected when your body is susceptible to it. To check if this was indeed happening, they had to ask each other if their bodies were acting like barometers, or if something else was the matter. They used their bodies to *know-now*, to identify the nature of today's problems and to think of appropriate strategies to deal with them.

Interestingly, their bodies are both the problem and the *instrument* used to diagnose the nature of the problem. They produce knowledge when they need it, about the atmosphere and about themselves. Van Leeuwen and his companion need each other's bodies to check what they are dealing with. Thus, they create a shared, practical and fluid way of physically being in the world, creating knowledge by and for bodies with extremely sensitive lungs. The illness here connects them to a caring community of people who share physical, emotional and practical capabilities, interests and difficulties, skills and strategies. These things are what fellow patients know *about* and *through* their bodies and from *sharing* this knowledge in order to test and check it.

Transporting knowledge

Mrs Smit's practical *know-now* (acknowledging and dealing with limits) has to be put to use in different situations. This is why the clinic started using webcams in follow-up care – to transport the lessons from the clinic to the home and other situations. Once patients had learned to observe and respect their limits under clinic conditions, they had to learn how to do this elsewhere. In theory, or as explicit *knowing about*, transporting this knowledge is not that hard. Anyone with an average memory can do it, and repetition brings the message home securely. It is different in the case of embodied knowledge. Explicit know-how needs translation, adaptation, reflection and training to become embodied so that it is effective and usable in varied situations. Everywhere, particulars need to be taken into account. No one book of rules fits all, and in any situation, no one skill always applies. If there are rules, these need to be sensed (Is this a limit?), interpreted and understood (Yes it is, and I have reached it because I overexerted myself) and obeyed (Now I should rest).

Back home after the clinic, patients sometimes referred to the 'laboratory situation' of the clinic where they had obtained theoretical know-how and put some into practice.

> Mr Bakker: There are so many little things you bump into. It's as if you have had 12 weeks of theory and practice, and when you're back home, you're thrown back on yourself. The transfer is really intense. It all seems so easy in the clinic. They show you how to do things. For instance, you learn to find a balance between exertion and relaxation. You should always exert, then relax, exert and relax, exert then relax. That's the balance. But at home, you have a date with X, an appointment with Y. And before you know it, you've slipped back into your old routines. You cannot learn new habits in only 12 weeks. In theory maybe, but not in practice.

Mr Bakker is talking about 'putting theory into practice'. The theory is not the problem here. Mr Bakker has an easy mantra for the theory ('exert then relax'). It is *enacting* the mantra that is causing him concern. There are many different situations and things to do in a day and over time. One situation is the physiotherapy class at the clinic. But it can also be 'back home', 'at work', 'looking after the children', 'shopping', or generally getting on with life as usual. The mantra, or theoretical know-how, has to fit varied situations. It is a directive for how to deal with the new and unexpected. It is not so much about *applying* knowledge, but about *living* knowledge in various contexts, shaping it 'in action'. Practical knowledge is about *doing* and *intervening*. *Know-now*, skills and propositions should enable people to act in multiple contexts.

Mr Bakker's story makes it sound as if the body 'forgets' the theory because various situations trigger different 'memories' of embodied routines. Mr Bakker slips back into his 'old routines'. *Situations* (and the people and devices within them) *have their own memories.*[41]

> Mrs Smit: Oh, you meet so many limits in life. In the clinic, it's easier to protect your limits because: a) they expect you to, and b) everyone has to do it. But back home, everybody is used to you just going on and on. That makes it harder. People don't realise what it means to have COPD. So it's harder at home than it is in the clinic.

Memories are inside and outside the body. In the clinic, many people were practising the same routines, and seemingly indefatigable carers kept pointing to matters of importance. To move practical knowledge from one place to another means making it present and memorable in new and different situations, even when those situations are not about disease but other things (shopping, caring for children, going to work, and so on). This means a re-organisation of practices outside the clinic to help people perform according to what they have learnt. The contextual expectations may stem from a situation with a healthy self, or a badly treated diseased self, and may appeal to competences that have faded away.[42] There is a great difference between *memorising* a mantra and aligning what it preaches with the demands, organisation and expectations of daily life.

In the rehabilitation clinic, the carers use *space* to create a different mind-set (or would its embodied translation be a different 'body-set'?).

> Caregiver: Green parks are pure invitations to go for a walk. People move less often because they get out of breath. But that's wrong. You should move in the right way.

People with COPD remember going for walks, but now walking only means trouble, getting hot and bothered and out of breath. So they stop going for walks and feel threatened rather than invited by the nice green park. The patients use the park surrounding the rehabilitation clinic to create new embodied memories, new routines, habits or skills. They learn to ride mobility scooters or train themselves to take breaks while out walking. But before new learning is possible, new imaginings must be unleashed. Scary parks must be transformed into attractive parks. This needs translation and transportation, and patients must discover, practise and arrange new fits.

Technologies and translation

Apart from mastering know-how and the skills to facilitate *know-now* and transporting and embodying them from one practice to another, there are also the bits of knowledge that patients get from doctors and devices.

This knowledge may not be 'ready to use' to improve daily life with disease. Before patients can establish routines, they need to develop fitting *know-now*, and to this end, patients need to make *translations*. As I made clear in the previous chapters, what devices do is not simply hidden inside their function. Users put devices to work and are put to work by the devices in turn. Remember the monitored patients in the last chapter? They could have interpreted their own measurements, but they did not. Instead, they left it to the nurse. The patients translate the direction that technology provides to make it useable and relate it to the concerns of daily life practices.

> Mrs Jarmus: You see, I had to learn to walk slowly, right from the start, walk very slowly. It doesn't come naturally to me. And then I used the saturation device and I noticed that after walking a minute, my saturation level goes down, or it drops below 90, and then I have to stop. So, well... a minute is not long.
> Interviewer: So you walk a minute and then take a one-minute break?
> Mrs Jarmus: Yes, that's it. But I find it so hard to put into practice! You have to stop in front of every shop window, look as if you're very interested in something, when there's nothing to see! Play with your car keys or whatever. And sometimes you just can't do even that. I have days when I can hardly get from the kitchen to the sofa.

Mrs Jarmus uses a device that measures the oxygen saturation level in her blood. She was told that 90% is the clinically relevant threshold; below that, saturation is too low to continue exercise without damaging tissues. But it is not enough to learn this fact in itself. Mrs Jarmus has to put this knowledge to use. She makes a first translation from *oxygen saturation* to *time*: after one minute of very slow walking, she should stop. The 90% saturation then becomes a directive to 'rest one minute'. Then another translation takes place; one minute's rest becomes in practice one minute of standing still. This takes place in public, in an everyday situation where people hardly ever stand still, on the street, and that makes it harder.

The body enacted by Mrs Jarmus is different with each translation of the saturation meter, and each body has its own troubles and possible solutions. The first body is a body with blood that contains oxygen that may sink to a level that is too low to keep moving without damage to tissues. This body becomes a body that should rest after one minute of walking. The body needing rest becomes a body that is visible to others and stands inexplicably inert in public places. This body needs to learn how to rest inconspicuously in public. A body too abstract needs to be adapted and crafted to turn it into a body that fits daily life or a body *now*. There are many different ways to do this. Giving Mrs Jarmus a mobility scooter would have led to a very different series of translations in her situation.[43]

Coordinating knowledge

The process of translation and embodiment opens up new sets of questions regarding *know-now*. For instance, Mrs Jarmus's use of the saturation device shows that the translations make it irrelevant to patients to distinguish between 'medical' and other matters. To call some interventions 'medical' could mean pointing to a particular phase of translation from the clinic to daily life. In the end, to patients, *any* intervention is an intervention in their daily lives. But translations are not always successful, even if they started as medical interventions. How does medical knowledge relate to other forms of knowledge? How do people coordinate knowledge from different sources?

Coordination practices, blurring distinctions

The case of Mr Hansen is a good example to show the blurring of medical and other forms of knowledge for patients. Mr Hansen used to be admitted to hospital regularly in an emergency ride with the ambulance. Nowadays he has a supply of prednisone and antibiotics in his medicine cabinet at home, so he can start treatment quickly if and when he needs it. His last hospital admittance was three years ago. 'When you get out of breath,' Mr Hansen says, 'the most important thing is to deal with your panic. That helps a long way.'

In theories of self-management, Mr Hansen has now obtained professional knowledge and has become a proto-professional, applying the knowledge and know-how of professionals for taking pills. And indeed, Mr Hansen knows that antibiotics cure inflammations. From the perspective of practical knowledge, however, Mr Hansen had to learn to develop knowledge that is practical in *his* situation now and in the future. He needs *know-now*, to find out *when* he must take the antibiotics, and if he must take them *now*. He must discipline himself to use his body as an instrument to sense this: he must not panic. He must decide if he needs to take a pill or do something else.

The distinction between medical expertise and lay knowledge loses its salience here, though one could say that Mr Hansen possesses the practical knowledge that, in its explicit form, used to be the sole expertise of his doctor. But as a mere proposition, it is abstract. For Mr Hansen it has become *embodied* knowledge that may be used by turning it into embodied, lived practical *know-now* that may tell him whether he needs antibiotics in this situation. As a mere proposition, it would be useless to Mr Hansen. Medical propositions need translation.

To complicate things, patients need to combine various forms of knowledge, medical and other, *even if these forms of knowledge seem incongruous* and *do not add up*. There were examples of this in the previous chapter, where Mrs Jansen and Mrs Jaspersen had to coordinate different forms of knowledge to deal with their disease. Bad lungs do not prevent walks in the park. Mobility scooters do not do away with inhalers. Monitoring devices do not stop fluid retention. Mr Griesemer was shocked to learn he was supposed to get better by seeing a *psychologist*.

> Mr Griesemer: I never knew you had to see a psychologist in here [the clinic]. I used to think, what's a psychologist doing here! It's my lungs that are sick. But, it's a very emotional disease. I never expected that. I'd reached this age, and never, up until one and a half, two years ago, I'd never ever cried, so to speak. Hardly ever. But these last months, aw, I'm howling like a baby. You see, you're not allowed to be jealous of healthy people, whatever. But you see people your own age out riding their bicycles. And you can't do that anymore. Well, that makes you feel really bad at times. I had to stop working. I don't want to talk about that. Still can't.

Mr Griesemer had a hard time dealing not only with his physical ailments but also with the sadness he felt, which his carers had diagnosed as grief at losing his past abilities. Mr Griesemer never expected this to happen to a body with sick lungs. He needed to adopt a new repertoire of knowledge, skills and tools to cope with this in daily life. Living with lungs that have given up meant finding ways to deal with tears and the sense of loss.

Besides involving knowledge and know-how from various medical disciplines, diseases tend to be entangled in practices for which no specialist knowledge is at hand. They are part and parcel of the daily grind.

> Interviewer: What did you learn in the clinic?
> Mrs Yildrim: Well, my family, eh... [laughs] I learned how to pace my energy, looking after the kids and the housework, too. You see, I always love my home to be spick and span, maybe *too* clean and tidy at times. I know that when I have a bad day, I should just ignore the mess. And the next day, when I feel well again, I don't do it all at once but keep on splitting the housework into little chunks. And with the kids too, I make it clear to them: this is what mum can do. And yes: mummy's now short of breath, and mummy just can't play with you. Not for a little while.

Here, it is not Mrs Yildrim's body that is the object of doctoring. She must develop knowledge, skills and *know-now* to cope with her love of a spick-and-span home and her energetic children wanting to play with her. She had to re-arrange how she did the housework and how she looked after the children. Again, a straightforward professional or lay, medical or non-medical distinction does not do justice to the complicated mix of relevant variables to be coordinated and reorganised here. Lungs, children and norms all play their part. And there were yet other problems to deal with, such as relinquishing work, ways of involving the spouse, and so on. Patients had to fit these matters and develop practical knowledge about them, often without professional advice.[44]

When helpful remedies occur in daily life, even if they start out as medical interventions, they do not have to retain a medical tint or texture. Practical remedies for dealing with COPD can be as unorthodox and varied as the problems faced.

> Mr Gregorus: The really hardest part was to accept it, and back then in 2003, I'd had enough. I didn't see the need to go on anymore. I'd had that many diseases, really, if there was one tiny little virus going round, I'd be sure to get it. Really. Then one of my daughters came in with that photo [he points to a photo on the table] of three of my four grandkids. She came in and said if I didn't know the meaning of life yet, I'd just have to look at that photo and then I'd be reminded. I don't know if it helped me through, but it's still a very important photo. [laughs]. It's holy, that's why it's in pride of place!

The picture 'works' for Mr Gregorus, enabling him to not give up on life or succumb to despair. The photo is an 'effective' intervention, although it would be nonsense to organise a clinical trial around photos on tables, even if it proved to be a life-saving remedy in Mr Gregorus' case. Disciplinary boundaries are useful for professionals and patients. Nobody would want to be given a pill that has not been thoroughly checked or undergo a merely experimental operation by a creative surgeon. The patient, however, faces the task of arranging input from different disciplines in a meaningful way, even when the input is contradictory. Is it despair or inflammation? Will it need a pill or a photo? How to combine written-off lungs with the attitude that allows one to keep moving? Patients do the work of coordinating this knowledge – if all goes well, with the help of their clinicians. The patient's position shows incoherent forms of knowledge, unlike within a medical discipline. Patients jumble many different logics relevant to daily life together in finicky practices prone to change. This demands impressive *know-now* and the ability to improvise in order to find ways of making this knowledge practical and thus supportive of living with COPD.

Unhelpful knowledge, translation failures

Translations between particular forms of knowledge and liveable daily life are not always successful. Medical practices may be counterproductive, as Mrs Thie points out:

> Mrs Thie: That doctor, the substitute doctor, he said [imitates accent], 'Well missus, it won't get any better than this.' Well, that gave me the jibbers! At Lungs [hospital department] they are so pessimistic, they don't give you much hope. So you've got to be optimistic yourself. Because if you listened to them... Of course, I know I'm ill and my lungs are very bad. But if you don't get over it and think, 'I will cope', well, if you don't do that, you'd die of misery.

Another patient called the lung function test 'incompatible with life', as if its message was: with this poor lung function, you are already dead. The fact that their lungs were not going to get any better scared patients because, in the shape of a statement of fact about their body, it gave them no handholds to organise life sensibly. If she accepted the proposition about her lungs, Mrs Thie would 'die from misery'. What *did* help her was knowledge that could be made useful – with or despite her damaged lungs. Mrs Thie did not shy away from the *truth* of the diagnosis ('I know my lungs are very bad') but from the implied pragmatics of this fact. As an intervention in daily life, it was counterproductive. It had no meaningful translation and improved nothing.

Let's now compare information on lung capacity with information that will help you cope with the difficulty of showering when you are out of breath, as Mrs Jacobs describes here.

> Mrs Jacobs: When you're done with the shower, well, you towel off [demonstrates drying her body and her hair], but she [her webcam friend] said: 'You can put on a bathrobe and wait till you're dry, you won't catch a cold'. That takes no energy, but drying yourself does! You have to learn to think like this. What would *you* do: after a shower you grab a towel. But now I take 15 minutes. The rollator is near the door, I bring the phone, in case someone calls. I take it easy and recover with my bathrobe on. Dry up a little, then put on a little deo, pat a little cream on my face, and then I dress. And I shower in the afternoons. I lie down for an hour or so, and shower after that.

In contrast to the knowledge derived from lung measurements, knowledge about bathrobes and towels is directly useful to daily life, even if it means changing the drying routine and no longer showering in the morning. The difference is not about empathy, or that towels are not *medical* solutions but about pragmatics. The advice can be tested and used at once. Instead of translation, it just needs a little rearrangement to put into practice, and instead of a depressing interpretation, it supplies positive instruction. As a form of knowledge it is provisional (it may work for Mrs Jacobs and her friend, but not for somebody else). But it is ready to be tested and close to everyday practice.

However, even when advice is practical, translations of various types of knowledge do not always succeed. Sometimes, the body will just not cooperate.

> Mrs Peters: I feel too young, and that makes it extremely hard. You want to do so many things, but you just can't anymore. The body says, stop. I was in good shape. Physically, I was already fit, but in the clinic I got even better. My arms can still pull an incredible load and my legs can push tremendous loads, and everybody working in the clinic was really happy with that. But then I'd think: What good does it do if my lungs don't work. What's the use?

Patients work on developing muscle tone in the clinic, and for many this meant their overall condition improved. They were more capable of walking. For Mrs Peters, however, more muscle power did not lead to walking longer distances or less breathlessness. Cooperation between the body of muscles and the body of breath had reached its limits.

At other times, patients did not translate practical knowledge into daily life practices because they did not want to give up the things they found important. For instance, in a session on self-care in the clinic, the patients had to list all the domestic activities they would normally do when they expected visitors.

> Caregiver: 'Have you all chosen the things you would or wouldn't do?'
> In reply, everyone says their home must at least be tidy when visitors come.
> Mr Fransen: 'I'd take the vacuum cleaner and clean up the mess, even if it means I'd be knocked out when the visitors arrive.'
> Mrs Pietersen agrees. 'The house should be dusted, vacuumed, the dishes done and the floor should be mopped. It is impossible to think that my visitors would come in to a pigsty, that's not how it should be.' She adds, 'And when I'm visiting someone else I always look to see if their house is clean. It's how it is, and how it should be.'
> Mr Fransen: 'I'd die of shame if my house was a mess. I'd do anything, even if I had to crawl over the floor with the vacuum cleaner.'
> Again Mrs Pietersen agrees.

The patients in this discussion value cleanliness over fitness. To them, it is out of the question to show visitors a house that is not clean. Dealing with disease is one thing among many other important things in life. People with COPD have to coordinate different problems and values in life. In doing so, they may make decisions that do not fit a medical logic, but they are rational from a different perspective. Concerns about children, not wanting to stand out in social events, or taking on too many tasks were among the reasons patients gave for neglecting their bodies. These trade-offs were unfortunate but unavoidable in a life with chronic disease.

Knowing patients

My analysis of bodies, medical practices and practical knowledge show how problematic it is to simply put professionals and patients directly opposite each other, as in expert versus lay, clinic versus home, knowers versus believers. Nor does it make sense to equate their knowledge as the same as in the policy on expert patients and studies of patient movements. It would be a loss of potential as well as an underestimation of the work patients have to do if scholars and patient activists would not ask questions about their knowledge or only focus on matters of power, such as staging patients as consumers. Instead, the analysis showed the complexity of using and developing practical knowledge in the daily life practices of people with COPD.

Difficulties of *knowing-now* and the complications arising from transporting propositional knowledge and directives across situations create this complexity. This requires embodied skills as well as a talent for improvisation. Patients need *translation* processes to turn different kinds of knowledge – such as knowledge from devices and specialists – into practically useful knowledge that enables living a liveable life with disease. There are no guarantees for success. Translations of harsh medical interpretations are problematic, and there are disobedient bodies and competing values. The complexity of putting medical knowledge to use helps us to understand patient 'incompliance' not as ruthless sabotage but as the difficulty of translating knowledge to fit daily life practices and combining it with other matters of importance. Medical directives cannot be lived by the book, simply because lives are not books but an accumulation of practices.

Added to this complexity is the variety of 'laboratories' or scientific disciplines involved. The patients must combine physiotherapy with medication management; they need to sort out entanglements with peak flow meters and embarrassments; tears and panic attacks need to be treated with training in breathing techniques, with kindness or domestic wisdom. The analysis pointed out that separating medical knowledge from more homely forms of knowledge is not very useful in daily life; both are interventions in daily life practices. However, the disciplinary boundaries do make sense to establish the effects of treatment. Patients may exchange and test the more homely tricks for dealing with disease far more freely. Practical solutions may not be helpful to everyone, but the real problem is that they *travel* badly. They do not easily fit medical specialisms. Nursing and physiotherapy could be the exception, but not all people with COPD have access to these disciplines. Homely solutions travel especially well when patients care for each other. This is an important lesson for developing future health care practices and policy.

Practical knowledge and webcams

Patients use practical knowledge. The telecare devices may support or hinder this use, but whichever way, they shape it together with other technologies and medical advice. The webcam may give access to another patient's explicit knowledge. It may facilitate practices that arrange *know-now* for participants, sensing and making sense of events together, and practices that supply first aid and support. The webcams in this practice unleashed a caring community of patients and supported their sharing of practical knowledge. For a patient group with little 'voice' or prospect of therapeutic solutions, webcams and patients together provided each other with impressive forms of 'together management'.[45]

PART III

Routines and efficiencies

6 Zooming in on webcams

On the workings of a modest technology

Doing invisible work

The previous chapter discussed the important role that webcams play when people with COPD exchange and develop their practical knowledge. The webcam gave *access* to knowledge and directed people to *develop* practical knowledge together. However, in contrast to the monitoring device in Chapter 4, the webcam did not seem to do much to *shape the content* of the exchanged knowledge. Instead of specifically defining, say, deviant measurements as problems to care for, the webcams seemed to leave the definition of problems open to the people using them.[1] The technology was behaving modestly. But just how modest is a webcam?

In this chapter I look closely at the more hidden and seemingly less rigorous ways in which webcams *do* structure care and contribute to the process of fitting. The aim is to learn how this open, unassuming technology tames and structures conversations, albeit not deterministically. I analyse 'close-ups' of the webcam directing routines and perceptions in care practice, influencing what that care came to be about. I quote users' experiences and analyse how both users and researcher observe the workings of the webcam. How does the webcam help create particular situations and experiences? How does a webcam 'work' in the practice of people with COPD?

Webcam practices

For the analysis I mainly use material from the rehabilitation clinic for people with COPD or asthma. Another set of material comes from a homecare organisation caring for patients suffering from severe COPD. In the rehabilitation clinic, patients volunteering to participate in the project received a computer with a webcam at home on their discharge from the clinic. They could use the webcam to keep in touch with their main carer in the clinic, the social worker. And, as I described before, they could also connect to the patients they had spent time with in the clinic as well as send email and surf the internet. The patients received the webcam for up to three months of follow-up care.

In the homecare organisation, the specialist nurse used the webcam to call on COPD patients every week. Here, there was no time limit on webcam use; nurses kept an eye on their patients as long as both parties thought it was useful. Besides contact with the nurse, patients could also have webcam contact with other homecare patients if they had a webcam too. At the time of the study, this webcam function was under discussion because patients were not using it spontaneously. Therefore, the professionals organised social meetings to acquaint webcam users with each other. I use the material from the homecare patients to demonstrate what webcams do with novice users – and the other way around.

Webcams in action

There are interesting studies on how webcams work. Sävenstedt, Zingmark & Sandman define the webcam as an invisible technology that does not influence human communication by itself.[2] They state: 'Transparency [in telecare via videophone] is understood [...] as a sense of presence and reality in the communication, even though it is mediated through technical devices.' The webcam is seen to offer a frame to communicate through, arranging what Sävenstedt and colleagues, quoting Knudsen, call *telepresence*. The authors describe telepresence as 'the subjective experience of being together with a person in one place when one is geographically situated in another'. The technology itself is invisible, something to 'look through' as if it were a window on the world. As with a pair of spectacles, it modulates but does not change what is there to be seen. It merely shows 'what is there' without influencing its object.

However, Chapter 4 showed that the webcam *did* change care and the object of care in various ways. The webcams helped to point out where to turn to in times of trouble. The webcam gave 'directions' for discussing both the nature and the solutions of problems with others. It changed the content of the conversations previously held on the telephone, for instance by helping carers and patients to 'see through' the embarrassment of reporting problems. In a psychiatric care setting for patients who fear social contacts, the patients see the absence of physical or material elements – such as smell, touch, the substance of the other person and their physical space – as a positive contribution to their care.[3] A webcam is not a transparent window on the world. It creates events that were not there before and would have been impossible to create without it. Webcam use builds new infrastructure, and it actively shapes care, even if the users are not aware of this.

'It is much more personal than the telephone'

How does the webcam shape care yet stay invisible? In general, my informants (patients and carers) used the webcam to have *personal conversations*. Both carers and patients praised the intimate nature of personal contact over the webcam. It outran the telephone by far, and people said it resembled 'real encounters' far better than a telephone conversation.[4] Communication partners repeatedly used the same phrase; they felt they were 'together in the same room'. Indeed, it seems they achieved the subjective experience of telepresence.

How did this close contact happen? Patients and carers often described the successes of the webcam by pointing to the *visual* element it added to the telephone's ability to transmit sound. They could hear and see one another. Being able to see the other person made it easy to respond and follow up on the other person's reactions; it made taking turns easier.

> Social worker: Conversations can get quite intense. How can I explain this...? On the phone, you've only got words and tone of voice. You can hear if someone is out of breath, if they're tense, having trouble breathing, or trembling. You know what it means if they compose their sentences in a certain way. It's different when you can *see* it all happening as well. Then you are closer, as if you're together, in the same room. Eighty percent of communication is non-verbal anyway. You lose all that on the phone.[5]

Although the list of non-verbal elements this carer can hear on the phone is impressive, he makes it clear that being able to look at your conversation partner allows you to be a better *listener* as well, because listening is a visual practice as well as an acoustic one. The non-verbal communication that webcams enable makes conversations more personal than on the telephone. Seeing the other person allows you to 'read' the listener better, you can see the listener doing just that: listening.

> Social worker: Take the two ladies I chat with [on the webcam]. It should be follow-up care, but is it? No. They simply have lots of problems. And I listen to their stories and nod understandingly. I keep quiet, I'm more of a sounding board [*praatpaal*] for them. That's quite a different effect from what the telephone allows for.

Obviously, nodding quietly would be ineffective in a telephone conversation since it involves a gesture instead of words, something visual and not a sound. Because both partners can see each other and react to what they see, the webcam can tune and relate interactions. Personal conversations 'fit' the way care is delivered through the webcam.

As mentioned before, the webcam helped social workers and nurses make their care more effective. They could see if the patients were not looking well, even if the patients were embarrassed to 'confess' this and said they were fine. Regular contact, strengthened by the intensity, reinforced the treatment. It could stimulate patients to work on their treatment plans or keep the intention to 'quit smoking' on the agenda. Patients also used the webcam for chats and distraction, to get their minds off their illness. It was important that their conversation partners knew about COPD. Then patients were saved the judgmental stares of the ignorant.[6] They felt recognised and respected by fellow patients, whereas they felt misunderstood by people who failed to acknowledge their invisible disease.

Webcams intensify concentration

Webcam users set and shaped all these tasks. Besides making conversation partners mutually visible, what did the *webcam* contribute to the intensely personal experience of conversation? How did it help shape this experience? The first thing to note is that the webcam seemed to *concentrate* conversation.[7] Talking on the webcam demands more attention than talking on the phone. You can do other things while you are on the phone, with mobile phones you could be anywhere when someone calls.[8] On a webcam, it is different. You have to attend the 'meeting' at a specific location – that is, at the computer. You have to prepare for the meeting, and sit in a particular position to stay in frame. Moving out of the camera frame cuts the contact at once. There is less distraction from peripheral events. Participants concentrate on their task and can only do other things as well if it is not a problem that the other witnesses this.

Interestingly, this concentration could be relieved in specific situations. For instance, two patients sometimes took up domestic work during their webcam chats.

> Mrs Van Houten: I had Jane on the webcam once. And I says to her: 'Jeez, you're putting yourself out!' So she says to me: 'Yes, I'm doing the ironing as we speak and why not? After all, you can talk and knit at the same time!' [This is a Dutch saying to encourage people to continue work while talking.] All these little things are nice. It's different contact from when you only phone someone every once and a while. It's far more cosy [*gezelliger*]!

It would be very impolite for a patient to do the ironing while conversing with the carer. But it is permissible for experienced webcam users in the informal interaction of friendship. It took place in variation to more focused and serious conversations.

The concentration in serious conversations also has to do with the way people look at a computer screen. The screen invites fixed gazing. Sävenstedt and colleagues measured the amount of time conversation partners spent gazing at the screen during video conversations. In a care setting, conversation partners spent 92% of the total time looking at the screen, whereas in direct conversations the percentage spent looking at the partner is around 50%.[9] This is a huge difference. Staring fixedly at the other is an artefact of webcam use. Moving out of the frame or diverting the eyes too long would mean you are breaking the contact.

Intense gazing is tolerable because webcam users do not look each other in the eye directly. The usual angle of a webcam makes people watching the screen seem to be casting their eyes downward. Thus, webcam users can stare at each other on the screen, but not directly into the eyes. This would be intolerable in encounters in the same space. Looking at someone's face for 92% of the time would feel very uncomfortable. It would be aggressive and too intense. Encounters in the same space contain many opportunities for participants to shift their gaze while still staying in touch. These encounters also *demand* that those present do so.

Gazing enhanced the concentration of activities, and so did the *framing of the webcam shot*. With the webcam mounted on the top edge of the computer screen, the camera angle frames the face and the upper body. The shot is steady: you cannot move much, or you would put yourself out of the frame. Thus, the webcam creates an *exemplary face-to-face encounter,* it being even more about faces than encounters in the same space. Apart from faces, the webcam does not present much else to look at. The things surrounding the computer – as well as the computer itself – are either invisible or irrelevant background clutter. This iconic face-to-face-ness excludes surroundings, other body parts, scents, handshakes and coffee cups. The frame of the webcam image sets a fixed stage for focused personal conversations.

Breaking the intensity

Where participants were friends, the intensity was often broken by the lightness of the chatter in webcam contacts; they showed more of their homes or they showed objects made or deemed important. It seemed that when the webcam partners were friends, there was no need or desire for intensity in all conversations. They did not have serious talks all the time. A chat could be just the thing to get away from your troubles. It was okay to reveal more about yourself, your home and your private life.

> Anne: One day I was chatting with Sandra [a fellow patient], and my mother and father came in. And Sandra said: 'Well, let me see them a bit!' So my mother sat down at the computer, and I said, 'So, this is my mum'. You see? That was really fun. Another really nice thing was that in the clinic I'd been sewing a dress, for a wedding. Then the dress was ready when I was back home. So [her social worker] said: 'Oh, show it to me!' And I could, just by holding it up to the camera.

Patients who had become friends introduced each other to their family and friends, showed off things they had made and invited spouses to join the conversation. Thus, the patients experienced the friendly webcam visit as a live visit to the home, and the better the contacts were, the more of the home and one's private life could be revealed to conversation partners. It relaxed the intensity of the initial face-to-face-ness.

However, not all webcam users felt that seeing the other made the conversation more interesting. These two women were practising conversing by webcam in the clinic:

Greta and Miriam are sitting in the training room, each at their own computer. Greta invites Miriam to a video chat by clicking on Miriam's address. Miriam gets a popup menu on her computer screen, which needs a mouse click to activate a choice. She has to choose whether she wants to accept the invitation or not. She clicks 'accept' and with a squeal of enthusiasm welcomes Greta's image on her screen. The teacher shows them how to enlarge or reduce the image, by clicking on buttons or dragging it with the mouse. Both Greta and Miriam keep the image small. They are far more interested in the option to send text messages and busily try this out. Greta comments that she finds the image too big when it fills the screen. It distracts her from the text messages.

Because Greta and Miriam were 'socialised' using MSN (real-time text messages) – the MSN had unleashed and tamed them – they could ignore the image and concentrate on typing and reading. Webcam technology may *invite*, *seduce* or *facilitate* certain uses, but it cannot *determine* or direct them, or only specific elements of these uses.[10] As such, it remains a modest and open technology. However, if people can be tempted to use a webcam properly, as a visual communication medium, its main endeavour is to create closeness. The webcam helps to shape intimate and personal relations.

Together in the same room

In this context of care and support, the subtle workings of the webcam brought about and aided a typically personal conversation. The static position of the webcam, the framing of the faces and the gazing at the screen concentrated the conversation and gave it the characteristics of a serious talk. Added to the feeling of closeness was the shared experience of being together in one room – telepresence, as Sävenstedt and Knudsen call it. The phone calls used in follow-up care prior to the webcam could not attain this telepresence. On the phone, people were always 'fine!' The phone gives few clues that can help a carer confirm or contradict such blithe statements.

So, the webcam made both patients and carers feel as if they were in the same room together when they weren't in the same physical space. What defines the space you *are* in when you are 'together' but in geographically separate rooms?

> Mrs Jones: It's just so much more personal [than the phone]. You can see one another and... Yes, I have the feeling that a conversation lasts far longer; you tell far more than you would over the phone. You are closer to each other. It's like you're visiting the social worker, as if you're in the same room. You really have to make time for it.

Mrs Jones feels as if she were actually calling on her social worker, whom she 'went to see' in the clinic. Talking to their carers on the webcam, patients saw the space they shared as the social worker's office, even if this place was not the actual place patients visited in real life. In order to save on cost, the homecare organisation had set up one webcam centrally for all social workers to use. The patients, however, were used to visiting their social worker's office, and this dynamic did not change for them, even if the social worker initiated contact at the appointed time. Probably, established routines defined the space as 'the social worker's office'. The place of visit was, however, different for the caregivers.

> Social worker: On the webcam you can see the cigarette smoking in the background. If someone says 'I'm fine', you can see from the way they hold their body that they are not fine at all. When you can see things, it's easier. You can say, 'Your shoulders are bunched, are you really okay? Did you really get out of the house?' It [the webcam] is an extra aid to check quote-unquote on a person. You can see and talk about things.

Clearly, the social worker is observing the patient in the patient's home. It is as though he 'went to see the patient'. Social workers talked about *home visits* and watched out for relevant indications for treatment such as sloppy dress or packets of cigarettes lying around. The conversation partners did indeed achieve telepresence, the sense of being in the same room together, in terms of intimacy but not in terms of space. Each conversation partner met the other in a different room. Patient and carer met in the space belonging to the other. Their conversation constituted a *topologically reversed telepresence*: I am at your place, and you are in mine. Topologically reversed telepresence would be 'feeling together in one room, while physically separated and subjectively being in the place where *the other* is'. You are indeed in two places at one time, and not necessarily in the space where the other person thinks you are.

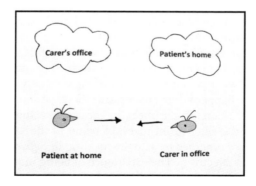

Figure 1 Topologically reversed telepresence

The topological mix of spaces was not fixed. It could change dramatically if patients felt the carer's gaze had become intrusive. Then, patients were no longer in the caregiver's office. They felt watched, spied on at home. This is *topologically congruent telepresence;* subjectively, both partners are in the physical space occupied by one partner.

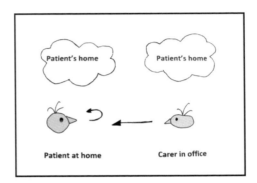

Figure 2 Topologically congruent telepresence

As you can see in the second figure, the direction of the gaze changes. For topologically congruent telepresence, both people are in the space belonging to one. One is 'looking in' from an unspecified elsewhere, the other is fixed in their own geographical (and emotional) space. When this space is the home, telepresence is experienced as more intrusive than when one visits the other elsewhere. Note that placing both in the carer's office is rare; this would make the carer the object of observation.

Apparently important to evoking a *positive* feeling of telepresence is that the space must feel safe for the task at hand. 'Gazing out' provides a position of control and activity, whereas 'being gazed at' is a far more vulnerable position. The fuzziness of the space where befriended patients meet each other confirms this. It is topologically reversed, switches between congruencies or between congruence and reversed spaces. When showing something off or discussing one partner's problem, they were in the place of the person either showing or revealing something. Chatting away, they could be anywhere. When both were ironing, they were visiting each other's place. How this game with space is enacted in different contexts is a matter for further research.

What does it reveal about the webcam? Again, the webcam does not determine what happens but creates specific experiences that are not usually possible when people meet in the same actual space. Mixing spaces allows the feeling of intimacy, of being in the same room, even while the intimacy emerges by actually meeting in *different* places, objectively as well as subjectively. The experience of being in the same room – that is, in the home of the patient – could be threatening for the patient when the one 'looking in' was the carer. How unassuming is this for a

ZOOMING IN ON WEBCAMS

modest technology? Even though feelings of intrusion are striking, the webcam does not *create* them. It enables these feelings to arise by creating the possibility of changing space.

Trust, familiarity and intrusion

If webcam conversations created intimacy, intimacy was a *precondition* for developing satisfactory webcam conversations as well. Patients regarded webcam contact with a strange carer who did not already know them as useless.[11]

> Mrs Green: That social worker has been my supervisor for 12 weeks, so she knows all my ins and outs. She knows the plan and what went on when I was in the clinic. If it had been somebody else, somebody I didn't know, it wouldn't have worked, no way. If someone doesn't really know you, they first have to get into your whole story. It just doesn't work. Only, truly, with your own social worker. They can say: 'We decided on this, this and that in the clinic, and you had these problems here, so how is it going for you now?' You'd never get that with a social worker you don't know.

Seeing and being seen on the webcam by an unknown person did not make sense, because the added value of being able to see one another did not pay off if the other did not 'know your whole story'. Patients had become experts on their lives and disease and had nothing to gain from general directions. They had plenty of that in their regular care. They needed detailed knowledge about their lives and bodies if follow-up care was to be of any real help. Intimacy or familiarity brought knowledge and tools to interpret a particular individual's situation (*know-now*).

> Mrs Nicholson: When I go to a sports class for people with chronic disease, I see my coaches once every two weeks. They don't know me at all. I find [the rehabilitation clinic] more important. You get feedback from somebody who's known you a long time and who has far more knowledge about COPD.

Patients talking to a new social worker reported that they were not happy with their webcam contact. It had no added value. The social worker could not 'see well' because they were unfamiliar with the way patients might look and behave when in or out of trouble. Their 'clinical gaze' was superficial, even if expert in general matters of COPD. It was tuned to a generalised patient, not to the individual.

The patients experienced the familiarity of the carer as very positive or even as a *sine qua non* for webcam contact. Familiarity had, however, its downside as well. The informed gaze, tuned perfectly to the individual patient, could also be experienced as especially and effectively intrusive.[12] The carer was not just an anonymous and objective observer or 'Big Brother'. He – or rather, she, to continue the gendered metaphor – was a well-informed 'Big Sister' (nursing sister) who not merely kept an eye on the patient but also knew what to watch out for due to intimate knowledge of her patient's personal ins and outs. In contrast to unfamiliar observers monitoring by camera or a monitoring device, Big Sister's experience and knowledge of individual traits and particularities ensured reliable, targeted registration of what was going on. Observing her patients, Big Sister could be an even better judge of their situation than the patients themselves.

> Mrs Strand: When I talked to her [the social worker] the first time, I was rather ill. She noticed and so she said: 'Really, if I were you I'd call the hospital now.' So I did and I was admitted. So then I said to her: 'Thanks a lot!' It's not that I want to hide from it, but yes, maybe I hadn't noticed how bad I was myself, so there you go!

The observer was right to connect what she had seen to Mrs Strand's asthma. Although the outcome was inevitable in due course, Mrs Strand disliked the fact that her social worker had suggested she be admitted to hospital before she had reached same conclusion herself. Worried others who 'keep an eye on you' may be intrusive, especially because they know you so well and are thus authoritative in their perceptions and suggestions about what to do. Indeed, 'being seen by the social worker' could be a major intervention.

But Big Sister could also be *wrong* in her observations.

> Mrs Strand: One disadvantage [of the webcam] is that she can see you. Yes, as far as they [social workers] are concerned, that's good, of course. But last week she said: 'You look very tired.' And then I thought: Grrr! [laughs] I had good reason to look tired, it was because my child was ill. Over the phone she wouldn't have seen that!

Knowing the caregiver and being known to them may imply intimate forms of accountability. Yet the gaze of the observer is fallible and needs confirmation from the one observed.[13] The examples clearly show how powerful the intimate gaze is. Mostly, patients regarded the clinical eye, with its thorough knowledge of COPD as well as their personal situation, as very helpful. However, the webcam brought this well-informed gaze into the home, and combined with the intense contact and a topologically congruent telepresence, it may become threatening and intrusive. Carers with the capacity to turn indications into symptoms with scary medical consequences stare at you in your home. A webcam has the capacity to support and strengthen intimate relations, but the device also permits what patients experience as abuse of this intimacy.

ZOOMING IN ON WEBCAMS

Building on existing relations

Relations between webcam partners have to be close if webcam contacts are to make any sense at all, and if they were not, the patients did not experience webcam contacts as helpful. Patients strongly abhorred having webcam conversations with people they had not met before and thus did not know at all. They were unanimous about not wanting to connect with people they did not know. One patient said she disliked being visible even symbolically to these strangers through the webcam system.

> Mrs Munichs: What bothers me, with MSN you can be online while your status displays 'offline'. But with the [webcam], you can't do that. When you switch the computer on, anyone [on the webcam network] can see straight away that I am online. Once I was called straight away, the very moment I went online. I don't like that. I didn't know what to say to this woman, I didn't know her. But I couldn't switch it off [the sign that she is online]. And to decline an invitation [for a video chat], that's not easy. It sounds so mean: 'I don't accept the invitation'. So I talked to her anyway. I would like to see when someone goes online, but I don't want to be online myself the whole day. So I leave the computer switched off.

This is a clear example of topological congruence, for Mrs Munichs feels she is being watched from *somewhere* in her private space. Being visible here means being exposed and available without being aware of who is actually 'looking in'.

It is possible, however, to change the rules for relating by webcam. The webcam does not give a fixed directive that 'one cannot meet strangers over the webcam'. Pappas and Seale show in their conversation analysis that, when used in care, webcam contact is a new form of communication.[14] Novice users have to negotiate the rules for using the new platform. In the homecare webcam project one woman *did* spontaneously call a stranger enrolled in the same webcam programme. Although they set out straight away to have a neighbourly chat 'over the fence', checking out mutual acquaintances and places both had visited, they negotiated terms of use for this new way of contact.

> Mrs Dantzig: Well, I thought, let's call Mrs De Bruin, that would be really nice!
> Mrs De Bruin: Yes, it is nice. We could do it more often. It's a solution, especially with this weather. [Heavy snow kept many older people at home in the winter of 2009-10.]
> Mrs Dantzig: Yes, I've been stuck at home for four weeks already.
> Mrs De Bruin: Yes, it breaks the day a little, doesn't it?
> Mrs Dantzig: Yes! You don't have to do it for hours, but every now and then, I think it is really nice.
> Mrs De Bruin: Yes, yes, yes.

[…]
Mrs De Bruin [rounding off the conversation]: Anyway, I did appreciate it very much when you called. And I will certainly call you back one of these days.
Mrs Dantzig: I think it's wonderful, too.
Mrs De Bruin: Not every day, though.
Mrs Dantzig: No, that's not necessary. But I think it's really nice I met you.

In this first spontaneous webcam encounter, Mrs Dantzig and Mrs De Bruin established new ground rules for how often and how long they would chat on the webcam and to what end. However, people who were not shy sometimes ran into trouble if they contacted people they did not already know. One woman thought that the aim of the webcam project was to support others by webcam. Therefore she started calling people, under the impression that the others were expecting her call. She had some unsettling experiences.

Mrs Sommer: Erm… I called a woman once and she said: 'I don't know you!' So she cut me off real quick. And one day there was this man, apparently he was looking for contact with somebody. I'd just spoken to the [home]carers, so I was sitting at the computer thinking, 'shall I play another game, or do something else', and then I got this man on the screen. So I said: 'Good afternoon, can I help you?' Well, he just sat there, staring, and didn't say a thing. Who it was, I wouldn't know. An old man, he was. And he had the device [webcam]. As for the rest, I don't know, I haven't tried to contact the others, because, well, I don't know if these people would agree to it.

Some people daring to try out the new platform were scared off, but most could not imagine what on earth they would talk about with strangers. They knew others were members of the same homecare organisation, but that did not give them enough in common. You would certainly not want to discuss your disease with a stranger.

Mrs Quest: I'm seldom in touch with the others [COPD patients, by webcam]. I don't have time, I don't really feel like doing it. What would you get? You'd both go: 'Oh, I suffer this or that, I've got pains in my arms and legs.' And then I'd think: I don't want to know, and they don't have to know this about me. Sounds crazy, maybe, but I don't want to burden other people with my ailments. These people [others in the project] have COPD too. And if they said: 'Oh, I'm so out of breath and I so need my inhaler!' Well, same here, but why tell everybody about it? Who needs to know? That's what I think, at least. Maybe others think it is wonderful to talk about that together. But as for me, so far, I don't need to know about other people's sufferings.

In contrast with the successful caring community that patients had established after their discharge from the rehabilitation clinic, some patients in homecare could not imagine getting anything out of a chat with a fellow patient. They did not know the others, were not friends, and could not imagine anything other than stilted conversations. The idea of exchanging practical knowledge was absent in this practice. Rather than knowledge, the patients expected to exchange 'complaints'. It comes as no surprise that they did not see this as an attractive proposition. It shows that friendship is an important ingredient for practices in which fellow patients may care for each other. If one shares nothing but a disease, there is no reason to become acquainted. Caring relations can only develop after friendship and shared interests develop first.[15]

Magnifying relational distance

The role of the webcam is to frame the relationship between its users in a particular way. People use webcams in situations where people who look at and are being looked at know one another and have a friendly, caring and understanding relationship. You may not know what space your conversation partner is in, you *do* know the space you are in yourself: this space is your own home.[16] This is especially clear when strangers 'intrude'. If there is no connection between persons looking at each other through the webcam, webcam communication does not resemble an actual meeting anywhere. It is instead a rude intrusion on personal privacy, or misplaced intimacy. If these visits bring about 'presence and reality in communication', they do so negatively, as an unwanted presence and reality that breaches the privacy of the home. It is awkward and undesired telepresence.

The webcam in this context thus changes *geographical* distance into a *relational* distance. It works best when the imposed relational distance fits the actual relational distance, for instance when talking to a friend or trusted carer. When relational distance diverges, the webcam seems to add to the strangeness or indifference experienced. The distance set by the webcam is then no longer appropriate. The stranger becomes even stranger on entering one's home; uninteresting or empty topics make contact even more meaningless.[17] This may be different for different people or different generations, or it may change if webcams become more common. It is clear, however, that the patients in the study did not want to invite 'just anyone from the phonebook' into their homes.

Framing and magnifying relational distance is quite an achievement for a webcam, even if its position in the home contributed much to this. Although there is space for users to ignore the relational distance, it almost never happened in the projects studied. The webcam made it hard to create a caring community out of members who did not know each other. Literally, they did not care. The webcam was better at facilitating relationships between people who did know and like each other. The webcam therefore did not stimulate contact with new people, especially because the space in which webcam users meet is in their respective homes. Meeting a new person would be less strange if it took place in a more neutral space.

What webcams do

Webcam technology seems open and unassuming, yet it influences and shapes care practices in very specific ways. It does this even if participants are unaware of the role this invisible technology plays in the course of a conversation. The webcam was seen to *concentrate* the task at hand. Because of the way a webcam conversation is set up, the way it frames the faces projected on the computer screen, it is difficult to do anything other than gaze at the screen. Framing makes distracting contexts disappear and forces conversation partners to focus on the conversation – and on the face rather than the eyes of the other. The result is the hyper-intense face-to-face topology described in this chapter.

It also concentrated the relevant tasks of conversation partners. If they were listening or caring, they were doing just that. Experienced webcam users could reduce the visual intensity the webcam provoked. They could chatter nonsense while ironing, they drew other people into the frame or showed (off) other objects, not just their faces. They revealed more of themselves and of their homes, but only on the condition that the relationship was intimate enough to allow this to happen.

Webcams *magnified* something, not merely in a visual sense, the way a magnifying glass makes things visible by blowing up their size or bringing objects closer. Instead, what the webcams magnified were *the existing characteristics of the social relationship between the webcam users*. The strange, unknown person encountered over the webcam became even stranger, maybe even scary or intrusive. A friend or trusted carer became even closer, as the webcam facilitated communication and support, benefitting an already good relationship. Hovering in the background could be 'Big Sister' and her close surveillance of the patient's home. Webcam conversation became indifferent and pointless when conducted with a neutral person such as an unfamiliar caregiver or a vaguely known fellow patient. There was nothing to talk about that demanded the intensity of a webcam conversation. And when there is nothing to say, the webcam mercilessly exposes this.

I described this magnification in terms of relational (instead of geographical) distance and space. Webcam-imposed relational distance might diverge from the relational distance between the persons meeting. This divergence relates to the location of the webcam; it was in the patient's home or in the caregiver's office, and this defined much of the relational distance the webcam contact imposed. A trusted friend or carer may visit you at home and may even let you feel a safe kind of topological congruence. A strange person 'looking in' may be a threat, because it places both the watcher and the patient in the patient's home. This space is too intimate to welcome a visit from a total stranger who gazes into the patient's domain from a nondescript elsewhere into which the patient cannot look back.

Places can switch fast. Compared to a 'physical' home visit, webcam visits skip the ringing of the doorbell, the hanging up of coats and other material and physical rituals of admittance. The webcam brings the visitor into the patient's room with a click of the mouse. There are no delays, no admission rituals. This poses no problems for a familiar person (and could even relieve the receiver from having to deal with muddy shoes), but for an unfamiliar person, actual relational distance would forbid the sudden demanding presence in the home, as the stranger would be 'in webcam proximity'.

Shaping care practices

The analysis showed the modest, unassuming but also forceful workings of the webcam. It showed that these workings are not fixed 'effects' of webcams. Webcam usage brought about a fragile network, populated by other users who adapt the frame, co-define the space they enter when they have webcam conversations or feel the power of defining space taken away from them. If all the elements of this fragile network are in place, the webcam can play its part in creating intense and intimate conversations.

Maybe it is a bad idea to speak of webcam *effects*. It could suggest that webcams have a universal functionality that is independent of place, unrelated to the specific characteristics of the user group and unconnected to the culture of use. It overlooks the diffidence of a modest technology. As an alternative notion, it may be better to draw out what webcams *are and are not good at* in relation to humans involved in particular (care) practices. This would both acknowledge the modesty of the webcam and take the creativity of its users into account, without erasing the actions of the device. A screen does not *compel* humans to stare at it; yet this is what they do because it is what humans do *and* because the screen seduces them into doing it. Listing the things webcams are good and bad at would define their potential or likely taming strategies.

Modest technology

Webcams are good at supporting – and intensifying – relatively close relations and in focusing users on the specific tasks they are trying to conduct. Webcams are unfit for tasks requiring physical touch or the bodily presence of people. Webcams are not of much use in the case of superficial contact, although this relates to the particular space in which people use webcams – in this case, the home. Webcams are good for checking on people but only in relations that permit this. However, because the webcam is a new technology in care, the ground rules for its use are under active construction. Different forms of fitting in webcams may well emerge. It may become feasible to establish new relations by webcam,[18] something the homecare projects will show in due course. It is safe to say that, if this ever happens, the relations will be friendly. That fits the context, and sustaining friendly relations is what webcams, in all modesty, are best at.

7 Economies of care

New routines, new tasks

What's in a routine?

So far, this book has documented many changes associated with the introduction of telecare, including changes in ideas about good care as well as the problems to target. As discussed before, *directives* come with norms and knowledge. Directives give pointers on how to establish a problem and how to look after it best. For example: keep track of your weight (directive) to check if your body is retaining fluid (problem), and if this is the case, the nurse will call you (directive) to intervene quickly (value). Directives become tacit or embodied *routines* when people no longer consciously follow them as prescriptions but live them as a habit, in ways they usually act. Knowledge and values consolidate to form the tacit rationale for ways of doing things. They become entrenched in the activities that enact them. In the above example, patients would routinely measure their weight even though they are not thinking about the reason for doing this.

Turning activities into routines is an efficient way of realising values and fitting facts. Not every activity needs extensive research, deep reflection or thorough contemplation. A further step to achieving efficiency would be to organise routines in a way that fits with their entrenched rationale. It would mean arranging routines such that embedded goals can be reached without wasting time and energy on matters of no (or less) importance to that goal – for instance, by abolishing superfluous diagnostic tests, reducing technical disturbances in webcam connections, and so on.

In this chapter, I want to show that a change in routine – for instance, by implementing a telecare device – does not always start with reflection on what new problems these routines will address or what values they implement. Telecare practices often show that the process has gone the other way around: routines change first, and the consequences take shape afterwards. This was the case, for example, when frequent measurements shaped disease as a daily changing process that needed quick attention. What it is that new routines implement may or may not be explicit. Here I want to explore how a change of routine has implications for notions of good care and how it impacts the organisational efficiency of care practices.

Routine efficiency

How can a mere change in 'doing' become so full of meaning and impli-
cation? A routine embodies the memory of something once learned, reflected upon, decided upon. As a fieldworker I have often asked myself
what I would have done in a particular situation that called for nursing
action. The answer varied between: 'I don't have a clue,' 'Quick, hide
behind something big,' or 'I might be able to answer this after a few
weeks of proper analysis, linking the singular event to notions of good
care and facts taken for granted on the ward, in comparison with other
practices.' If nurses took such a hesitant stance and had to reflect so
deeply before engaging in activity, that would be very bad news for their
patients. Routines embody (or solidify) professional memory and experience. *The nurse is skilled and knows what to do.* She can reflect on her
actions at the time or in hindsight and might judge that it wasn't the
best thing to do after all. In my experience, nurses are good judges of
their own behaviour. At the very least, they will know which course of
action to take or repertoires to choose from.

Routines link to *efficiency* in the sense that they make it possible to act
with economy, skipping the need for extensive reflection whenever
something needs doing. Efficiency is always part of the way in which
care is shaped and the other way around: any care practice has its own
form of efficiency. This is not a matter of mere organisation. Behaving
efficiently relates directly to the nature of the care given, because efficient behaviour aims to reach a particular goal.

A recurring example demonstrates this point. It is the complaint that
homecare services are organised as discrete technical activities within a
fixed period. For instance, helping a person to put on elastic compres-
sion stockings to prevent thrombosis equals eight to ten minutes of caring time. *Translating* care into manageable units is often criticised as a
way of *reducing* care to the activity of putting on stockings (rather than,
say, providing attention and signalling problems at the same time). Organising according to time units is, however, a way of creatively shaping
care. It fails because, to carers, care is more than 'putting in minutes'. It
will eventually fail for managers, too, because it is at odds with professional notions of care. Routines and efficiency are not merely about process and organisation, because these in turn are not only about routines.
They are about *specific* ways of bringing about something *in particular* –
one thing, not another. Like the telecare devices, routines shape what
problems are and how to solve them.

This is why changing routines in care, when introducing new telecare
devices, is so complicated. Routine change is informed by the nature of
local practices ('We have a Catholic tradition'), the goals set by local
carers ('It is important to visit our patients at home'), their managers ('I
want to put our organisation on the map'), the functionality of the device
('It cannot provide group statistics'), its relation to other devices ('I al-

ready have a computer at home'), and so on. It is an interaction between different variables, different logics even – some unknown, some evolving. Contingency and unpredictability are always elements of innovative practices. Routines may seem to be practical, mundane activities that are trivial in and of themselves. What could there be to taking a patient's blood pressure or sending a fax to a GP? I show in this chapter that there is a great deal to these activities.

To explore what routines do, what changing routines implies and what it reveals of the efficient organisation of care, I analyse material from *all* the projects to show that comparable things happen in each project. In an attempt to tame any possible confusion for readers, I start each section by introducing the cases used in the argument.

Telecare and efficiency

To trace the workings of routines or 'things done', let me discuss the ideal of efficiency in terms of the economic implications of telecare usage, as predicted by public discourse. Sources of the analysis come from my field notes, from newspapers and mailing lists, notes I made on policy developments, meetings with decision makers, and telecare conferences. The latter are often hybrid gatherings where consumer organisations, telecare providers and care managers as well as the occasional researcher meet. These happenings are often promotional events, which makes it easy to analyse the changing promises and solutions of telecare in context – the latest hype.

Telecare promises efficiency. More precisely, telecare has at least two efficiency promises with very different implications for the organisation, the goals of care and the problems to solve. Different logics define the two efficiencies. The first promise is that telecare will permit efficient use of scarce health care *staff*. By *substituting* face-to-face contact with telecare contact, the gain in travel time alone promises greater efficiency. The associated ideal – telecare helps patients *manage themselves* – guarantees a reduced need for staff, with an even smaller number of professionals able to care for a growing population of elderly people with chronic diseases. And, as is common in economic reasoning about care: efficiency always promises to benefit a 'higher good'.[1] Here, the higher good is better quality of life for patients. Modern patients presumably prefer to manage themselves.

The second promise of efficiency fits the workings of telecare practices better as far as the analyses in this book are concerned. All the studied practices show that telecare use means an increase in the *frequency* of contact between patients and professionals. What is won in travel time (for patients or professionals) is immediately lost in the added frequency of consultations. Contact frequency changes dramatically from a consultation once every three to four months to daily contact and added telephone contact (health buddy, monitoring vital signs) or weekly contact (webcam). In this second form of efficiency, more frequent contact is the mechanism that makes care more efficient. This logic of *prevention* argues that increased contact frequency leads to better professional scrutiny of patients, preventing exacerbations and crises, while promoting a healthy lifestyle at the same time. Ergo, telecare reduces hospital admissions. This calculation concerns health care *costs* rather than the efficient use of *staff*, as it would demand more rather than less nursing power. The benefit for patients is obvious: fewer or no medical crises, and no emergency trips to hospital. The only worry is how they might die, eventually (but see below).

Both notions of efficiency savings – staff or costs – have very different implications for both the organisation and aims of care. Responsibilities and roles of professionals and patients differ greatly. Self-management ideals and reticent professionals compete directly with increased professional surveillance and passive patients. Moreover, both notions are *ideals* when compared to the current organisation of health care. These efficiency ideals confront health care practices in knowing yet other ways of doing things and professionals had other reasons for doing them. There was, for example, the importance attached to meeting patients in the same space or being cautious with medical interventions.

Efficiency in practice

How do the efficiency promises relate to real care practices? The notion of cost efficiency oversimplifies the flow of money between organisations. For example, it is unclear who will benefit financially. Many institutions may be involved, such as hospitals and homecare organisations. Reducing hospital admissions is attractive and would be an easy winner in any overall cost calculation. However, this could only happen if accountants bring the costs of telecare installations and the staff to make them work into the equation.[2] The homecare organisation or the hospital must pay for telecare systems and staff. In the first case, the homecare organisation invests but reaps no benefit from hypothetically saved hospital costs. In the second situation, the transfer of budget is also unclear. Reducing admissions means less income when beds stay empty, whereas the cost of telecare, the staff and technicians running the system demand immediate investment.

Both staff and cost-saving economies seem to take a bird's eye perspective, suggesting a household budgeting book for the nation as a whole. This move negates the complexity of the game of supply and demand played by various actors. There is no simple market with one party for supply and one for demand.[3] There are several sets of customers and suppliers. There are the professionals who need to make demands for telecare but do not actually make them.[4] There is the telecare industry that wants to sell devices but has difficulty accepting reluctant profes-

ECONOMIES OF CARE

sionals as their customers. They would much rather sell their devices directly to patients. The *patients*, however, have no purchasing possibilities whatsoever in this market, even though their representatives are much in favour of telecare developments.[5] Individuals may only agree to a system if their local care organisation happens to supply it.

Many organisations are watching their pennies. The expected costs and scarcity of health care staff is a political issue quite remote from the reality in consultation rooms or the concerns of the nurses caring for patients.

> Nurse in homecare organisation: The higher-ups in the organisation, they say it [the webcam project] needs to save us time and money, but we don't think this is the goal for us [nurses]. It could be an added benefit. As a professional I think it's important that people get good quality of care. Everyone has their own objectives in this project. It's up to us [nurses] to show that we can do it, at least for quality of care. You put things on track to improve care for patients.

Another unclear facet of the cost-saving story is the assumption that prevention will effectively *erase* disease exacerbation, but this remains speculative. An alternative chain of events is that prevention may postpone exacerbation to a later date in the lifetime of the patients. Preventive surveillance will improve their quality of life for some years and they may live longer, but the costs would still come at the end of the patient's life, on top of the costs of telecare. It is an intervention in quality of care, but an efficiency gain is unclear.

Even if the government were to attempt to reshape health care to allow for market dynamics, which supposedly lead to efficiency, telecare does not function like a market. The only way that one could look at telecare as a market is if one is content with the idea that 'there is no demand' from health care professionals and organisations. Yet this would gloss over the intricacies of a situation that is not really a market, and it would not do justice to the potential of care at a distance, an issue I address in the final chapter. For this analysis, suffice it to say that there are two notions of telecare efficiency in the debate on its introduction, whereas there are far more efficiencies in the implicated practices: the efficiency of singular health care institutions, of professional groups, of local organisations working together, of ways of living with disease, and so on. They all demand the arrangement of different routines.

Efficiency does not exist on its own and cannot be isolated from ideas of what care should do, who should do it and with what aim. Should patients form caring communities as they did after leaving the rehabilitation clinic for COPD patients? Or should they be pushed to manage themselves, even if they are accustomed – and prefer – to care for others? Efficiency alone, in the shape of savings in costs or number of staff or other aims unrelated to care, can never be the final objective for health care reforms without the reasoning becoming absurd. If saving costs was the only concern, one might as well give up on the whole idea of having a health care system. Instead, it would be better to ask *what kind of care* is desirable, how it would fit existing efficiencies, what roles professionals and patients should have and how to organise it at an acceptable cost in terms of money and human resources. Managers must formulate the goals of care first before turning to the question of how to organise care efficiently.

The place of caring

Routines are sticky things. Different notions of what care should look like, what it should aim for and how to do this best tend to stick to routines and interfere with other ideas of good and efficient care. The next case moves away from policy debates and onto homecare. In this homecare organisation, the project manager is trying to implement webcams. The case demonstrates the difficulty of changing existing routines. The project manager did not expect to run into the trouble he encountered. He thought telecare would just be a new tool (webcam) that nurses would use to achieve what they were already trying to achieve. He did not expect the webcam to change the very nature of care.

> Project manager: The nurse should join in the [telecare] system. I think she should come to see the telecare technology as a building block in the care process, as an extra means at her disposal to solve her care issues and reach her care goals. No more, but, mind you, no less either. It's something extra, to add to what we had before, to the care process we've been used to for hundreds of years.

The project manager looks at the webcam as a means towards an end, where the end does not change if the means do. The impact of using webcams on the working routines of the nurses, however, proved something else. The project took place in a few villages and suburbs of a city in the south of the Netherlands. Homecare patients received a computer with a touch screen at home. They can use it to play games online or, via the Service Centre, to win prizes. Users can access local services on the system, watch 'church TV' and contact other users (which, as I discussed before, they rarely do). They can also contact the homecare organisation. The idea is that embedding care in other useful and nice things to do with the computer makes access to care easier. The system intends to reduce the loneliness of older people in the neighbourhood and help them stay at home safely, but with a low threshold to mobilising care if they need it.[6]

Theoretically, there are two ways to contact the homecare organisation. Patients can call their local homecare team, or the Central Calling

Point (CCP). CCP workers are situated elsewhere and are connected to all users from all the locations. The CCP is important in getting patients to use the system. CCP workers may call patients on the 'Good Morning Service'. In these sessions, they discuss the patient's plans for the day and possible problems, but the contact can also be just a chat. The aim is to get patients engaged in using the telecare system.

The project manager encourages the local teams of nurses to use the telecare system in their work. And this is what my research assistant, Esther Leuthold, interviewed him about. The first step, he explained, was to introduce the new technology to the nurses and have them reflect on the possibilities it might have for them.

> Project manager: We [the project team] organised a workshop, so that they got to know what it is. And then we brainstormed together on what it could mean for the care processes we're engaged in. Who among your people [patients] could work with it or would like to try it? Then we put the webcam equipment in their offices for them to play with. [...] But with one team, we didn't take enough time to follow up their work and keep encouraging them to use the webcam. It seems it slowly bled to death, the device just stands there now, gathering dust. They [the team] use it every now and then, but only very occasionally. So we said, we should pick it up again, give some training, do project meetings, case meetings, and bring it back to their attention. So that they don't forget it, so to speak.

Similar to patients trying to remember their new lifestyle rules, the neighbourhood teams also have their own memories, routines and practices. Reminding nurses to use the webcam in their daily work is, however, also a reminder that routines must change. The webcam will only work if it gains a useful place in the work and goals of the carers. This takes time and effort, including special training, playing, thinking together and reminding each other, according to the project manager. Merely placing the technology in homes and offices is no guarantee that people will use it at all or even sensibly.[7] Devices only function in relation to other things – the power supply, the internet, managers – and their users.

This is one of the difficulties for the manager: opportunities may seem clear to him, but the nurses need to change their practices to apply them. Existing practices are full of 'memories'; these routines have served their purpose for some time and are kept alive by many actors and devices in their particular alignments. Participants rearrange old practices to make new devices work. This is hard if the people who have to work with the device do not perceive the need for it in the first place and require instruction to become aware of its potential usefulness. Even when they are convinced the technology has some good use, it is hard to change practices and tame devices in work routines. Working routines are material, embodied and relational.

Reshuffling space

There were various routines in the homecare practice, and some were more easily established than others. Establishing the new Central Calling Point was easy. It provided new jobs that people could apply for, and it operated from a new office. It was different for nurses who spent their working days out in the neighbourhood making home visits. The paradox is that if they used the webcam, they would have to stop going to the patient's home. They could care for patients from the office, making the actual space occupied by the patient irrelevant to care. But this space was not irrelevant to the *nurses*. To use the webcam they had to move *away*.

> Project manager: They could use it to make an arrangement with a patient. They'd say something like: 'I'll call back later to see how it went.' And then they'd continue their tour of the neighbourhood and when they got back to the office, they'd contact the patients they needed to reach. If they play with the system like this, they'd get experience. I hope that they'll do it more systematically, give it a steady spot in their services. That they'll say: 'Before, I went out there to help a person start the day, get them out of bed, get them to wash, dress, have breakfast', that kind of thing. They will replace all that with webcam contact. The nurses may not perceive this as a particularly efficient move, considering where they usually are.

The manager's logic of economic efficiency was about 'substitution' or 'saving staff'. The difficulty, however, was the place where the nurses gave their care. Moving it from the patient's home and into the office is a radical change that feels paradoxical when you want to care for patients. It means having to leave patients alone in order to care for them.

Moving care into the office brought another spatial difficulty. Having the carer's webcam located outside the patients' homes interfered with the communication technology that homecare teams were accustomed to using: the logbook in the patient's home. Several professionals call in on patients using homecare, including cleaners, assistants to help people get out of bed and wash and dress, as well as the nurses who tend to medical matters. All professionals write their reports in the logbook, something that is not possible when giving care at a distance. The distant carer simply cannot write in the log kept at the patient's home.

> Project manager: This is really complicated. The log is our form of reporting. 'I was here and did so and so'. You can tick a box if you want to point your colleagues to more information in the dossier. Say: 'I prepared the medication, but the stock will only last another three days. Can you order more pills?' This is the job of the First Responsible Nurse (FRN). The log is the most reliable and complete system we have. It's kept in the patient's home. The GPs, if they come to the house, they also report that in the log. But the CCP is at a distance, and CCP staff cannot write in the log, which

means if they have something to communicate, they have to call or send an email to the FRN. I'm dreaming of setting up an electronic record or some other shared document system available on the internet.

The situation is indeed complex. All carers used to share their position in the home of the patient. Take away one important set of carers, and a communal communication system runs the risk of collapsing. Changing the working routines not only concerns the actual use of new technology but also the logistics of care – in this case, of communicating with other professionals. Nobody had foreseen this in the brainstorming sessions on the potential role of the webcam in homecare for patients. One change leads to another, and the chain of events is not always easy to oversee, let alone supervise and manage. Routines are not easy to change. They remember, they make people remember and they interconnect. It is not easy to swap logbooks, Stick-It notes, emails and telephone calls for an electronic record that as yet does not even exist, let alone call this efficient. The hoped-for efficiency lies somewhere in the future, and its shape is still unclear.[8] This makes it hard to create the changes needed for the webcam to function acceptably and to inspire the nurses. Rather than improving things, it created new problems for which, at the time of the study, there were no solutions.[9]

Different technology and tasks

The policy debates on telecare efficiencies demonstrated the close relations between care routines, notions of efficiency and what care came to mean. The project manager's problems with implementing webcams showed how caring routines form a network of related activities, technology and tasks that is impossible to change without changing the entire network. The next case analyses a phenomenon in *all* the projects studied. Not only the quantity but also the quality of the nursing tasks changed when nurses started using telecare. I will illustrate this with material from the different practices.

A frequent complaint was that new telecare technology added extra *administrative tasks*. Nurses found themselves looking after the telecare system rather than their patients. This was also an artefact of the research that accompanied the new practices. Research needed extensive registration of patient data. The nurses conducted and collected registrations, and this was yet another unanticipated change in their working routines.

The heart failure nurses in the hospital came to 'share' their patients with call centre nurses who monitored the outcomes of the heart failure patient's daily weight and blood pressure measurements. Protocols defined the tasks and responsibilities strictly, but the heart failure nurses in the hospital felt that their patients had disappeared from their practice. In the meantime, they remained responsible for them and had to keep the patient record for the call centre up to date. The record for the call centre was a duplicate of their own administration, and the trial evaluating the monitoring project also used these data. Care for a telecare system and its evaluation are quite different from care for patients, even if the tasks are related. The hospital nurses would have preferred the extra work of following up on the monitored values themselves. They disliked merely doing the administrative tasks.

> Heart failure nurse: Well, it's my personal opinion but... my colleague agrees. In that other study, we were the ones checking the patients. This time around [the monitoring practice study], I see nothing. So I have no connection with [the study]. I have to tell you: I never look at the programme, at the weights and such. We used to do that when we were in charge of the project. But now, we get an email from [the call centre]: 'Patient such and such has put on 800 grams and would we please discuss this with the cardiologist.' Well, our cardiologist says: 'I don't want anything to do with it anymore!' He [the cardiologist] gets called for a patient who's gained 800 grams in a day! We know these patients well. With some, you'd think, 'That's not ok'. But with others you'd think: 'It will be better tomorrow.' You see, this is a very small hospital, we know the patients really well.

At the same time, the nurses from the call centre were troubled by the difficult route they had to take in order to induce a small change in a patients' medication, particularly diuretics. The call centre nurse had to call the responsible heart failure nurse, who in her turn may have to talk to the cardiologist. The heart failure nurse then had to phone the call centre nurse, who in her turn called back the patient. This demanded an elaborate coordination and the call centre nurses felt it did not do justice to their professional capabilities or meet the need for efficient care. They felt they could be responsible for diuretic medication, just as the patients themselves sometimes were. Careful, explicit task allocation made sense in terms of liability and responsibility, but it made less sense from the viewpoint of nurses more interested in patient care rather than in administration.

The oncology nurse using the white box in palliative care experienced a comparable problem with elaborate administrative tasks:

> Oncology nurse: Well, you can imagine, before the white box I would say to a patient: 'I'll call you after the first chemo, and if you're worried about something, you can call me.' Now I have to explain the workings of the white box, input their data into the system, put the copies in the file, and take the file in and out of the filing cabinet. I have to read the results of the patients' answers every day, and see what is new. Call someone, do this or that. Fax the GP. It all takes time. And the coordinator wants to know everything for the research: 'Oh, we don't have the diagnosis for Jansen, and here

we need a little detail for Geerts, date of birth. And did you get this form for Klaasen?' We have a control group, they 'just' fill in the questionnaires, but they need to be in the system as well. And well, I have to look it all up, go to the cabinet, take out the files. That's how it goes. [...] It's just, it's so much extra work. Make a new file here, noting details there about patients and writing timesheets. And also your research, that again costs time! It's all really small things, but added up, it's a lot. And it's all time that's not spent on your patients.

The oncology nurse did not work with a call centre. She ran the system with the help of the technicians and the service provider maintaining the system, and she did the administration herself. Much of this work dealt with distributing information on the system and recording data for the research tangled up with the project. Adding an extra device to a care practice meant adding a new node in the information network around the patient; it meant storing incoming information and collecting data for the research, and keeping other professionals informed. The nurse tacitly took on this extra burden, if only because no one else was available. No one had anticipated the effort needed to make the system work.[10]

The rehabilitation clinic also had administrative problems. There was a discussion about assigning the telekit (computers with webcam) to patients. At the start of the project, staff assigned the telekit to patients they selected themselves, but later this changed into offering it to as many patients as possible. The reason was the wish to do a quantitative study that would objectify which group of patients the telekit could help.[11] In practice, the new goal resulted in many dropouts and telekit offers to relatively healthy people whose care would not improve anyway. For instance, during office hours it was hard to reach by phone, let alone by telekit, the relatively fit people who had gone back to their jobs.

The new assignment strategy revealed many patients unwilling to participate for a wide range of reasons: not enough space at home, no desire to have an extra computer, about to move house or not wanting to make the disease too central in their lives. Here the needs of a projected future practice (evaluation research) interfered with the ways the clinicians put the telekit to use. This changed the way of offering the telekit from a way that fit a *care practice* to one that fit a *research practice*. The research practice tamed the telekit so differently from the way the clinicians had tamed it that the clinicians often considered it unhelpful.

The homecare specialist nurse for COPD patients provides a last example of the changing tasks for nurses, highlighting the complexity of organising information flows and administration. Here, the nurses used both the white box and a webcam.

Homecare nurse: Now we work with four screens [points at the computers]. There is one for the white box, with its own network and database. And then you have one for patient records, our own information, including listings of who we call, and the care dossiers. For the white box you need to put the info into its own system. But if patients only use a webcam, then you have to put it in a different patient record, because you need to put your information somewhere. Then there is the contact screen [to talk to people] and the call-in screen [for incoming calls].

Several systems depending on different networks and databases meant that the nurses had to align a complicated series of devices and checks. As the oncology nurse said, these were 'all the little things'. The nurses performed these tasks for the greater good of patient care. Again, nobody had anticipated the extra work of collecting data and distributing information. All this comprises a new form of care in nursing practice: care for the telecare system and its evaluation. Telecare does not in itself create efficient work practices. Efficiency needs to be organised in and around them.

Interpretation routines

The next case is from the rehabilitation clinic for patients with COPD and asthma. It demonstrates how working routines around the same technology may become confused because technology – the computer with webcam (telekit) – has various identities. What the technology is and how it is supposed to support the aims of care practice differs, as do routines to use it efficiently. However, these differences in identity are tacit, and routines became mixed up tacitly. At the time of the study, managers, technicians and carers were discussing the future of the telekit. Their deliberations over the potential uses of the telekit held opposing ideas on what care is and what it should be about that troubled its terms.[12]

The telekit had two identities related to different treatment goals and sets of routines for efficient use. The first identity relates to the goal of *guaranteeing the effect of the treatment*. This turned out to demand very different usage routines compared to the second notion of what the telekit should do: *provide a window on the world*. For these different treatment goals, the identity of the telekit became a *digital umbilical cord* connecting the patient to the clinic, or an *inhaler* providing the 'puff' to get on with life. The metaphors come from the clinic staff, although they did not use them consistently.

The telekit as an umbilical cord

When the carers formulated the purpose of the telekit as 'consolidating the effect of the treatment', proponents intended it to help patients develop 'adequate behaviour' to cope with their illness. This meant that patients had to put into practice what they had learned in the clinic. The telekit directly relates to, and stands in the service of, the work done in the clinic. Here, the metaphor for the telekit's identity is 'the umbilical cord' that attaches the patient to the clinic and allows them to be 'fed' more of the clinic's wisdom. In this view, contact with the principal carers – social workers – was central to telekit usage. The principal carer was supposed to check on the patient, discuss their problems with them and encourage them to take the steps laid down in the treatment plan they had made together in the clinic. Contact with the social worker guaranteed the continuity of the work done in the clinic.

Contact with fellow patients would serve the same purpose: to bridge the gap between clinic and home by giving advice on how to cope. Three months of computer use was thought to be sufficient to reach these goals. The use of email and internet was a more ambiguous aim in this scenario. Patients were supposed to become *independent* of the clinic and its devices, with the telekit remaining in the realm of the clinic. If patients wanted to go on using the computers after the umbilical cord was severed, this was encouraged (and indeed trained for) in the clinic. However, the clinic would not be providing the hardware. People would have to buy their own computers, just as they would have to join their local sports clubs and rely on care from their 'own' specialists and home carers. Hence, email and the internet was seen as ambiguously both part and not part of the treatment.

In the end, the proper way to deal with umbilical cords is to *cut them*, when the attached one has other, more 'grown-up' resources and means to feed themselves independently. This is a specific notion of treatment as 'a temporary intervention by professionals'. The treatment effects must be consolidated, but ultimately the professionals are supposed to make themselves superfluous. Treatment has to stop, and people have to learn how to fend for themselves with the help of their local carers. They have to cut themselves free of the clinic.

The telekit as an inhaler

When the purpose of the telekit was 'to provide patients with a *window on the world*', the telekit mainly became a device to actively continue the tasks set in the clinic and get on with life better. One problem patients have, for instance, is social isolation and loss of meaningful activities; they do not have much to do with their day. Many had trouble leaving the house, and they learned solutions for this in the clinic. Patients could tackle problems by establishing a more permanent social network with fellow patients. Fellow patients could become friends or close acquaintances connected by webcam and provide enduring support and company.

Internet and email usage was important in this telekit framing. Patients need to employ both in their routines as structural ways of seeking entertainment and keeping in touch. The internet connection supported such services as home delivery of shopping, membership of online gaming, entertainment,and social media. The telekit thus became a structural part of the social, practical and emotional life of patients, permitting many different contacts after the carer from the clinic had stopped seeing them. The device supported patients in building their new world.

In this case, the telekit is a permanent aid rather than a temporary lifeline to the clinic. One of my informants described this form of the telekit as an *inhaler*, a device that COPD patients use continually to counter breathlessness. When the telekit is like an inhaler, patients are dependent on it. That makes it rather cruel to withdraw the device after three months. It would be like giving a person a wheelchair – or indeed an inhaler – and then taking it away even if the need for it has not disappeared. People should not *emancipate* themselves from the device but rather use the telekit structurally, as useful and dependable technology.

Of course, as in the former scenario, the clinic's care would not be permanent. Here, too, patients had to cut themselves free of the professionals, even though some thought this was indeed a pity. However, the treatment would not be limited in terms of time. It would be ongoing as patients used the new device to reshape their world, making it part of the everyday muddle of getting through the day and facing new problems. The telekit functioned as an inhaler rather than as an umbilical cord.

Routines and identities

The two identities of the telekit meant two sets of routines, implying two ways of organising care at home efficiently. The double identity of the device and its use were not explicit. Both scenarios were present at the same time, with the carers unaware of the differences. That they held different views on *treatment* was something they had not come up against before. The technology simultaneously materialised and separated the different goals that the carers could accommodate before. On the one hand, treatment should have the effect of helping people find meaningful connections to the world. On the other hand, practising what one has learned during treatment is a way of engaging with the world. The telekit differentiated these aims by separating the different sets of routines that patients needed to employ to achieve either goal.

In the daily telekit operations, the different sets of routines were tacitly present, with one or the other in the foreground. On a theoretical level, the two ways of caring and using the telekit were different, but in practice they were mixed up, muddling discussions and complicating practices. The case shows that planning routines is complex because people may have different tacit understandings of how they should use a technology and how to use it efficiently. Implementing a device has unpredictable consequences for working routines. But even if the telekit complicated the different goals of treatment, both goals are still valid.

Both treatment effects – consolidation as well as adding meaning to life – are important and overlapping assignments for patients. Efficient organisation of care practices, particularly innovative practices, needs to accommodate and coordinate different logics of care and thus align different sets of efficient working routines.

Old or new routines?

My last example is from the practices using the white box in the care practices for people with heart failure and in palliative care. This example shows how people use old and new logics of interpreting situations to make a device work. The old logic involved routines for interpreting information delivered by patients face-to-face, relating information to the patient's individual situation. In contrast, the new logic involved new routines of interpretation through coding, according to general protocols for heart failure or palliative cancer patients. In Chapter 4, I discussed the coding in the context of patients and nurses making individual exceptions to the rules imposed by the white box. Here I analyse the nurses' interpretation routines.

Even if the patient's answers were coded, nurses still made sense of this information by using their clinical routine of relating information to the situation of individual patients. They did this to make the information meaningful to them in terms of knowing what the matter is with patients – in particular, how they should respond to the information provided.

Field note
I am looking over the shoulder of the oncology nurse to see the data she has received from patients on the white box. The red, amber and green alerts are listed on top. There is a red mark for a woman who hasn't slept well for three nights running. We discuss what this might mean. 'You don't know what it means,' the nurse explains, 'so you have to look for clues on whether to call the patient to ask, what's up?'
Another patient has a red mark registering the lack of sleep, and there is yet another bad sleeper on the list. Now this is a pattern! We realise that the previous nights have been extremely hot for Dutch standards. This is a good enough reason for not sleeping well. The nurse has discussed the remaining alerts with the patients concerned. She knows what it means if a particular patient feels 'a bit less well than yesterday'.
A lot of data, still in the nurse's head, is related to the situation of individual patients. One patient reports that he is using different medication from the prescribed one, and this gets a red alert. The nurse knows he uses homeopathic meds that are not relevant to the treatment in the hospital.

The white box generates a lot of information, but what does it all mean? The heart failure nurses tackled this problem by reading *all* the answers and establishing their own evaluation criteria, calling up patients when they were in doubt. This meant an impressive multiplication of the amount of information the nurses received, compared to the four visits a year that used to be the standard. Answers came in every day, taking approximately 2 minutes per patient per day to read, not counting the follow-up calls.

The two logics for assigning clinical relevance, following codes or relating answers to the remembered context of individuals clash here. If the nurses followed the code logic, they would have to make many unnecessary calls. If, however, they had to contextualise data, the workload of the nurses would expand even more than it already had. The codes would be efficient if they provided fewer 'false-positive' alarms. In the palliative oncology practice, the team tackled this problem by continuing to tinker with the question protocol to remove any ambiguities. They also added a question asking patients whether they would like the nurses to call them if a coded answer signalled an alarm, mobilising the judgment of the patients. Keeping samples of patients small also facilitated the use of contextual information.

This example shows that new routines do not simply *replace* old ones. Carers needed old routines of interpretation to make the new ones function at all. Thus, new routines are not necessarily *better* than old ones, and the new ones may even depend on the old. In terms of efficiency, the extra new work is again obvious. How these tensions are resolved once telecare becomes routine is a question that the developers of these projects will need to show in due time. So far, telecare has established a change in the quality of care rather than a reduction in cost or improvement in efficiency by saving staff.

Treacherous routines

Routines are not isolated acts. They are consolidated values and knowledge. Routines are a prime way of enabling efficiency; they make it unnecessary to think about every act. Routines or devices tacitly embed values and knowledge, and time revealed the implications of changing them. Because of their inconspicuous and tacit nature, the 'density' of routines may remain hidden for a long time. Routines tend to link to other routines and devices, enacting different notions of good care and types of problems to care for. Sets of routines enact particular logics of good care, fitting notions of efficiency. The analysis showed this when analysing the notions of efficiency in the public debate on telecare and the different use practices of the telekit.

The interdependencies of routines made it difficult to change them: changing one element in their organisation – for instance giving homecare nurses webcam tasks in the office – had implications for the organisation of care and communication between different carers. The task of the carers changed, but not always in a way that suited their wish to care for patients rather than the telecare system. The nurses performed the administrative tasks that were needed to make the telecare system work, to align the telecare administration to their own and that of other professionals and researchers. Nobody had foreseen this extra workload when the implementation of telecare was under consideration.

Unpredictability was a recurrent characteristic of implementation practices. Differences in tacit understandings of the purpose of a device explained this unpredictability, as did the clashes between sets of working routines, as was the case with the interpretation routines of the nurses using the white box and the nurses collaborating with call centre nurses. An efficient organisation of care practices needs to create space for this unpredictability as well as for the differences between sets of routines needed in care. Chapters 4 and 5 illustrated the different routines patients could run into, because they had to enact the advice of different medical specialists and combine this with other things that were important to them. These chapters also stressed the importance of *improvisations* in reacting to new situations. Care cannot exist as a routine practice only.

Efficiently organising messy practices

A more efficient organisation of care practices is thus not merely a matter of organising routines more tightly but also of aligning different forms of efficiency. Efficiency is a concept that is as variable as notions of good care or terms framing what is wrong with patients. Attempts at rationalisation may interfere with efficiencies in current practices, creating a mess rather than efficiency. This mess will eventually result in new working routines and improvisation strategies, but what shape they will take is hard to predict. This analysis demands more respect for existing routines than is common in innovation practices. New routines are not always better, and sometimes new routines only work with the support of the old ones. Whichever way, new routines need to build on the old by gradually translating, adapting or aligning old and new routines. Designers of telecare can never anticipate the complexity of care practices, which involve many norms, contingencies and forms of knowledge, nor can they build it into the technology. The slate for the design of devices is blank, whereas practices are not.[13]

CONCLUSIONS

On studying innovation

8 Innovating care innovation

The politics of innovation

By way of conclusion, this chapter draws out the lessons of my analysis for innovation practices in care and suggests ways to study them and argue about them. The general conclusions about the workings of the telecare practices are embedded in this chapter. The last section entitled 'Discussions unleashed by an uncontrolled field study' draws out some general lines on the use of telecare in health care.

Back in the introduction, I described innovation in telecare as a process occurring between the market and the soapbox. The Dutch government's idea was to place care in a market context where competition among care providers – reinforced by assertive care consumers and rival health care insurance companies – would lead to efficiency and quality improvement. Active consumers (patients) will not buy care they do not want, and they are unwilling to pay too much for the care they *do* want. Hence the market provides a new political arena separate from parliament. Instead of voting, participants in the market state their opinions by (not) buying health insurance and care services. The consumer patient has become a political actor.

However, the dialectic of quality and efficiency has not emerged in telecare developments. Although the government, national patient and consumer organisations and health insurance companies all promote telecare for its assumed quality and efficiency, the market seems to have run into a brick wall on this issue, with all participants pointing at each other to make the next move or accusing each other of preventing the next move from taking place. Random projects survived, while many others did not. Project survival rates said more about business, marketing and prestige than about how the public[1] – especially (potential) patients and professionals – would define good quality care or living a good life with chronic disease. Knowledge on the workings of telecare was virtually absent.

What did emerge was a lot of soapbox posturing, with those for and against telecare spouting forth either unsubstantiated promises or imaginary hell holes in an attempt to move telecare development forward or stop it. Proponents pushed the telecare hype to create a demand for sales, while opponents warned of the dangers of cold mechanical care. Besides the telecare industry, however, it remained unclear who stood to gain from telecare – patients, professionals, care organisations or financers? – and who should pay for it all. If all the concerned parties are potential customers, all have diverse interests that do not always fit harmoniously together. The development of telecare in the Netherlands has come to a standstill despite a number of pioneering projects and a few spectacular failures.

In this final chapter, I explore a policy development method for innovation in care, including telecare, that takes a different stance from the soapbox or market approach, although it may accommodate both. My method looks for ways of bringing *knowledge* into the debate, rather than settling on wild hopes or dire warnings of how telecare will or will not work. I reflect on a different sort of *research* that actually delivers useful knowledge on novel telecare practices, that engages the parties concerned and their practical knowledge while granting more space to the actual telecare users – patients and professionals. By identifying concerns that emerge in practice rather than imaginary ones, this research considers normative issues more productively than the market or the soapbox permit. The research design aims to *fit* innovative telecare practices better than conventional research does.

Before outlining this 'fitting research', I shall recapitulate on the *object* it should establish better fits with: innovative telecare practices. I show why traditional quantitative research methods – the randomised controlled trial (RCT) and, more common in this context, its less robust family of related research designs – do not fit this object. I analyse three misfits and one more general concern about conducting research.

The object of research: innovative telecare practices

What innovative care practices have I described?[2] The three parts of the book showed that implementing telecare changed the *type of problems* that participants addressed. For example, telecare could shape problems as deviations in weight and blood pressure or as indistinct worries demanding further inquiry. Telecare also changed the *ways of addressing* problems. While patients measured their vital signs daily at home, nurses supervised their interpretation. Previously, both the organisation of measurements as well as their interpretation had been the responsibility of the patient. Another example of how telecare changed the way problems were addressed is the webcam. Patients used webcams to name and frame possible remedies, mobilising the experience of other patients rather than professionals. The webcam allowed an exchange of practical knowledge that had been mostly absent in patients' practices.

Besides defining problems and the remedies to address them, the telecare devices influenced the *values* that participants pursued in order to make care *good*. Prevention by early intervention became a value of monitoring practices, replacing the values of medical caution, self-help and patients' initiative. Webcams stimulated not only the exchange of patients' practical knowledge but also the potential for mutual support, shifting responsibility from local professionals to patient communities. Care aims to improve daily life with disease, and devices aim to achieve this goal as well, even when notions of improvement differ greatly. If a device is to be helpful, patients, nurses and devices have to establish fits between them, shaping problems as well as good care. My analysis showed that these changes were often tacit, as they began with a change in caring *routines*. A change in the *frequency* of contact, for instance, had great consequences for understanding a problem and the best response to it. Moreover, the new routines needed to relate to the old ones and interacted with them in various ways. For instance, the old practice of meeting patients in the same space continued alongside new telecare practices.

These changes and interferences as well as the ways users behaved made the nature of the established fits unpredictable.[3] Innovative telecare practices – the object of the research in this book – were complex practices still under construction. Building plans changed along the way as a necessary part of fitting in new devices. Seemingly sensible theories about care and the workings of technology were proven wrong, again and again.

Unpredictable results were a core characteristic of innovative practices. Whether certain devices in care practices lead to self-management, to supportive social networks or to the neglect of a device depends on many contingencies. This is a matter that the participants and their devices are still busily working out between them, in circumstances they may or may not be able to influence. Spelling out these contingencies provides insights into how to possibly influence future practices. Yet, however different they were, the outcomes contradicted both the promise of improved efficiency and self-management as well as the nightmare of alienated patients.

Research that does not fit

Fixed variables and unpredictable outcomes

If innovative care practices involve the process of crafting new outcomes, research designs that need predefined fixed outcome variables will not fit. Such research designs gloss over the most important characteristic of innovative care practices. This means that RCTs and their family of research designs are not particularly fit to study innovative practices. State-of-the-art evaluation research *does* define its variables at the start of the study, to evaluate the effects of well-defined interventions on well-defined outcome measures. Quantitative researchers recognise the problem of evaluating telecare practices because interventions are difficult to stabilise, involving activities of devices *and* users. Researchers complain about suboptimal designs of telecare studies that make it hard to assess the effects (see Chapter 1). This is a first misfit between quantitative evaluation research and innovative care practices. A more fitting design should permit insight into the processes that (re)name and (re)-frame goals and problem definitions.

Subjectivity and practical knowledge

Patients and carers develop practical knowledge in innovative care practices, including knowledge about normative problems and ways of dealing with them. Quantitative evaluation studies, however, cannot use this knowledge. This is the second characteristic of innovative telecare practices that does not fit classic evaluation studies. Learning how to fit in their devices, users engage with the ups and downs of doing so and in the process reflect upon normative issues that unexpectedly emerge along the way. Classic evaluation studies, however, cannot tap productively into this experience. Fitting research might well do this, but how?

The norms of the RCT family of research designs consider practical knowledge and normativity suspect. Classic research does not use practical knowledge because RCT methods are supposed to provide knowledge that is *more reliable*. These researchers regard practical knowledge as *subjective* and as providing disturbing factors rather than helpful insights. A basic value in the foundation of RCT and related designs is to strive for *objectivity* to replace subjectivity, and to use procedures that guarantee it, such as double-blind research and the random selection of patients.[4]

But is practical knowledge subjective? To answer this question, I take a closer look at how subjectivity is understood in the context of research. In twentieth-century research, subjectivity has two influential meanings. The first is *interests*. RCTs were designed to control the pharmaceutical industry.[5] New drugs should not be given to patients without satisfactorily establishing their workings and possible adverse side effects. The RCT guarantees that industry interests will not influence the outcome of research.[6] The methods employed should make it impossible to influence results, even for 'interested' researchers.

The second meaning of subjectivity relates to the *use* of scientific knowledge. Quantitative research designs aim to ban the arbitrary (subjective) administration of treatment. This stems from the tradition of evidence-based medicine (EBM). The motivation for EBM is to guarantee that patients will not get a particular treatment only because their doctor has a particular *liking* for a particular course of treatment, but because there is *evidence* that this treatment *worked* in an acceptable percentage of comparable cases. EBM puts objective knowledge in the place of doctors following their own fads or hobbies, treating their patients with favourite therapies. RCT results thus *correct* the doctor's practical knowledge and provide ways to discipline it. Research-derived knowledge is free of self interest, fads or any other subjective factor related to individual doctors.[7]

Interestingly, and quite contrary to the idea of banning subjectivity, as I discussed in Chapter 5, there is a recent trend to improve medical research by engaging patients. Both goals – objective research and patient involvement – were reconciled by assuming that successful patient engagement depends on the agreement of both patients and medical scientists on what medical knowledge they should look for and what methods scientists should use to obtain this knowledge.[8] Unsuccessful participation, on the other hand, is attributed to the patients' lack of medical expertise.[9] Patients and doctors cooperate in their shared quest for scientific medical knowledge. Again, this does not put practical knowledge to use, and it is difficult to see how it could be done in a paradigm of research that aims to ban knowledge that is different from 'evidence' (probability) of effectiveness.

My analysis, however, showed the differences between practical and scientific knowledge, both for patients and for professionals.[10] These differences were not about *subjectivity* or *interests* in contrast to objectivity. The differences were, first, between the *aims* of practical and scientific knowledge. Practical knowledge aims to help treat individual patients, whereas scientific knowledge attempts to create and accumulate knowledge based on probability calculations.[11] Second, there were differences in *developing* and *accounting for* practical and scientific knowledge. This is the difference between RCTs and meta-analyses, on the one hand, and the hands-on work of treating *this* patient on the other. In the hands-on case, carers must apply their experience in comparable cases and integrate it with the technology they use while translating medical knowledge and concerns about what is good in this particular case. In the meantime, clinicians keep track of the patient's response and adapt the treatment if it does not have the desired effect. Practical (hands-on) knowledge and scientific (theoretical) knowledge have different pragmatics, different time frames and different relations to truth or certainty.

Placing subjectivity and objectivity in opposition does not describe the differences between scientific knowledge and practical knowledge. This becomes particularly clear when one considers ways and possibilities of developing and transporting practical knowledge, making it more robust by sharing it in critical analysis. It might be worth trying to *explicate* practical knowledge and critically assessing it, instead of banning it. This seems worth the effort when there is no other knowledge available because state-of-the-art scientific knowledge is unhelpful or uninformative. I will discuss the possibility of using and improving practical knowledge below and come back to the question of 'interests' and the truth claims of practical knowledge. But before I do, I need to discuss a *third* characteristic of innovative practices and a third misfit with state-of-the-art quantitative research.[12]

Interference with construction sites

A third characteristic of innovative telecare practices is that they are *sites under construction*. Ideally, fitting research would not hinder, disturb, or harm the construction of the innovations. This is difficult in state-of-the-art quantitative research because these designs need researchers to construct their *own* workplace to create the conditions for good research. Conditions need to be standardised, patients need to be randomly assigned to experimental and control groups, and questionnaires need to be filled in by carers and patients, and so on. In Chapter 7, I discussed the work the nurses did to collect data for research. Instead of caring for their patients or tinkering with the devices, the nurses were taking care of telecare administration and evaluation. Chapter 7 also provided the example of carers who had to offer a telecare device to all patients in the clinic, even when they knew the device would not apply to some patients. They had to include these patients anyway to allow research methods to establish objectively who would benefit from telecare and who would not. This directly hindered daily care.

Another example of research creating a competing construction site was the case of the white box in palliative care. There was no attempt at randomisation for ethical reasons and because of the small number of patients and the difficulties in recruiting them. This meant the results from the accompanying study were shaky, even with a control group in place. Here, good care was valued more than good research. The rigorous design of the RCT to evaluate the *monitoring device* led to nurses signalling mismatches between patients and research conditions ('It would have been something for Mrs Franken, but she's in the control condition'). The videos under construction during the study made it difficult to evaluate them. Researchers nonetheless collected data and analysed them.

The introduction (Chapter 1) gave another example of interference in construction sites in the discussion of the interdependence of research practices and the telecare projects they evaluate. The idea, of course, is to base continuation of the telecare project on the *results* of research. However, this scenario never unfolded. The telecare project depended on the *infrastructure* of the research so that it stopped when the research stopped. Researchers and nurses did not collect data anymore and the budget for the telecare project ran out when the budget for research did. In the long wait for the proper bureaucracies to process the results – bureaucracies that, indeed, found conclusions indecisive to warrant further investments – the telecare practice came to a halt as well.[13]

Hence, there are *two* construction sites – innovative care practice and research practice – that obstruct one another. Both sites aim to construct different edifices that sometimes support each other. At other times, one construction site emerges at the expense of the other. For instance, in the *research* construction site, carers *should not* tinker with interventions, or Mrs Jansen's intervention would have been different from Mrs Pietersen's. Otherwise, the research would evaluate different interventions and thus become useless. In care practices, however, adaptations were *improvements* – for instance, they softened the overly confrontational questions asked on the white box or adapted alarms that were not useful. The construction sites of care and research collide because of their different objectives, making it hard to combine state-of-the-art quantitative research with state-of-the-art care.[14, 15]

From subjectivity to normativity

So there are three misfits between RCTs and innovative care practices. RCTs cannot deal with unanticipated outcomes; RCTs ignore practical knowledge rather than use, develop and substantiate it; and the construction of randomised trials interferes on a practical level with the construction of innovative practices. I should point out a fourth interference that applies in general to any form of research. The discourse on objectivity obscures the fact that research designs interfere with their object in theoretical or conceptual ways. The designs themselves are fit to ask some questions but not others.[16, 17] Standard evaluation research can never ask how outcomes shift and change – variability can only be dealt with quantitatively, on scales of fixed variables. Scales measuring 'self-management' will never uncover 'feelings of safety', while the meaning of both terms – and their relations – cannot be clarified by quantification. Standard quantitative research designs are fit to evaluate relatively simple stable interventions in a context that can be controlled and standardised, such as for a drug trial.

You can trace the theoretical interference of research designs by analysing how the instruments and concepts used in the research shape the possible questions and outcomes. To be clear: interference is unavoidable and not wrong; no research is possible without tools and concepts. However, I would not frame interference as gradually encroaching *subjectivity*. That would suggest that researchers could and should avoid it, and that 'non-interference' is possible. Instead, I suggest opening this idea up to reflection and analysing it as the *inherent normativity* needed to say something about the world in research.[18] Here normativity refers to the articulation, the search for tools and concepts, or the naming and framing of the object of research, practically and discursively, foregrounding some facts rather than others. For instance, research may address vital signs rather than loneliness, may allow variables to change value or not, may ask open or closed questions, or create probabilities or develop practical knowledge.

It may be more constructive to argue about the *normativity* of scientific articulations than about interests or subjectivity. The latter two have a history of being 'bad' regardless of context. Instead, researchers could argue about *fitting* research methods and objects. How does the method shape the object of research and why is this acceptable? Does the method make relevant aspects of this object visible (for example: does it not learn about self-management when safety is the relevant variable in practice or does it help to understand the intricacies and different meanings of self-management)? Does the research not disturb the phenomenon it wants to study in such a way that the research studies a different object altogether (for example by lumping different use practices for the same devices together)? When is it best to count and when is it better to analyse practices?

One problem might be that the way the research names and frames its object belongs to the practical, tacit knowledge of *researchers*, since it is embedded in the machines and tools (questionnaires, interviews, blood tests, concepts) that are commonly applied in their discipline.[19] It may inexplicitly shape their practices as a tacit part of the history and routines of a discipline. Others – observers – may be better at articulating this. But even if researchers are not always aware, they can be asked to account for their ways of fitting in research methods and for the validity of their articulations.

Fitting research

So far, I have dealt with three misfits between quantitative evaluation research and innovative practices, and one concern with the normative interference any form of research makes in the way it frames or articulates its object, and whether or not a particular interference may fit with what you actually want to know. What does fitting research to innovative practices entail? Here is my list of norms needed for fitting research to innovative practices:
1. The research describes the processes that shape and shift the goals and outcomes of innovative practices.
2. The research mobilises practical knowledge, including practical normativity, without obscuring the situated and contestable nature of this knowledge.
3. The research observes and describes the practices concerned but does not disrupt the innovative work.
4. The research is sensitive to ways of 'naming and framing' or articulating its object and the consequences and 'fitness' of these articulations in relation to the aim of the research (in other words: aims and methods should be made to fit).

In discussing the ways of fitting research – I dub them *uncontrolled field studies* – I pay particular attention to the matter of 'interested parties', the status of practical knowledge and the potential to make uncontrolled field studies relevant for policy.

Uncontrolled field studies

Uncontrolled field studies are flexible forms of research that describe actual, innovative care practices where processes of taming and unleashing new devices (or new standards, new guidelines, etc.) have begun taking place with a minimum of disturbance.[20] The innovative practices may resemble the case studies in this book, even if calling them 'uncontrolled field studies' was never considered at the time of the study. Uncontrolled field studies in care are *uncontrolled* because it is not the scientists but the carers, the cared for and the other care participants who construct the research site by (re)constructing the site of care. They work with the devices and are the sources of relevant knowledge on what the devices do and what they do with the devices. Participants and their practices also shape the normative issues that are particular to their practice, even if one does not agree with the ways participants choose to deal with them. The participants of innovative practices are encouraged to interact with the telecare devices (by those in the innovative practice who find reason to do this), opening up their practices to research that describes the ways they do things and what that implies for living and working with a particular device. Innovative practices exist 'in the wild'. They already exist and do not depend on research projects that define their beginnings and endings.

How do uncontrolled field studies work? The researcher's task is to not disturb or change the work of participants and, by extension, the innovation. The researcher should record and analyse this work by asking open questions, observing practices, interviewing participants and asking them to observe their own practices. Then, researchers may *compare* results with: a) previously formulated goals, and b) the results of other innovative practices. Other involved and interested parties may then *discuss* these results.

Now I move on to discuss how uncontrolled field studies engage telecare users and the status of the knowledge these studies develop. By way of example, I describe some of my analytical results as a means of feeding knowledge on the workings of telecare into the debate on what forms of telecare are fit for whom and for what reason.

The influence of users

Uncontrolled field study can include concerned parties in several ways. On the first level, the concerned are identified because they are involved in the innovative practices, not by having a voice or a budget but by getting the 'space to act'.[21] On a second level, rather than merely asking for their opinions, the uncontrolled field study engages users by an analysis of their *positions* in the innovative care practices. What positions for nurses and patients emerge, what are their possibilities, problems and responsibilities, and what should we think of them?

From buying, selling and voting to enacting innovations

Uncontrolled field studies analyse innovative practices as *situated* and *creative* practices rather than *deliberative* practices such as those of democratically chosen spokespersons in parliament or the *consumer* practices of buyers and sellers on the market. All involved in the practice *act*, and in doing so, all try to tame the others to fit their goals; they experiment with devices and the other participants to see if they can achieve productive ways of fitting. For instance, patients may try to nudge nurses into calling them rather than having to make a call themselves. Patients may refuse to use devices they do not like. They had already done this in the practices I studied, even when they were eager to 'help the nurse'. Old women who enjoy reading in peace and quiet *did* switch off a noisy device.

Telecare producers do not have the actual power to push their technology onto actual users (hence their anger and frustration), but they may try out their ability to *seduce* actors into working with their devices. They can do this by making promises, but it would be even more convincing if they tried to argue and demonstrate how their devices could be helpful. They could participate by adapting the devices to their users' needs. This would enrich rather than disturb the uncontrolled field study. Interests do not have to be *banned*; they are named and analysed in the study. If they are part of the reality of the innovative practices, it may indeed be a good idea to keep an eye on them.

Nurses and other professionals working with telecare devices are important actors in uncontrolled field studies. They are the co-constructors of the innovative practices, and researchers should not hinder them in this work. If they subvert the device used in the experiment, this should not be seen as a breach of protocol but rather as a creative attempt to improve care which deserves reflection. Tinkering could be encouraged by involving designers and technicians in the innovative practices, to adapt the devices to make them fit better with the aims and interests of the practices in which they are used. They may explore new uses for the devices together with the nurses, to make the devices work better.

This turns innovation into *creative* experiments rather than *standardisation* exercises, unleashing rather than taming devices and users, demanding curiosity rather than pointing at protocols and user manuals or making accusations of 'resistance' to 'proper' innovation or implementation. The study should take users' objections very seriously and explore them – if possible in comparison to other practices. One example is the nurses' desire not to replace visits to patients entirely with telecare. The merits of this claim deserve careful study rather than gratuitous appeasement acceptable to nobody. The logic of the uncontrolled

INNOVATING CARE INNOVATION

field study is as follows: if translations, tamings and unleashings must take place anyway to make things fit, why not encourage these activities and explore where they might lead?

Deliberations do not shape innovative practices. In innovative practices, actors craft their preferred positions by exerting their influence and trying to have things their own way. Patients beg to keep devices longer than intended, hand them in sooner or refuse to use them at all. Nurses find new uses for the devices and call their patients when they are in doubt. Instead of *arguing* about fit, the participants *create* specific forms of it. New interdependencies arise which can be described and which then enter the discussion on their desirability.[22]

Rest assured, innovative care practices are not totally anarchistic practices that go in just any direction as long as the innovation runs. In practice, this does not happen. The studies in this book show that routines, normativities and knowledge practices already fill care practice. It is hard work to establish the needed fits. Carers cannot do it any old way. 'Old' routines are never entirely abandoned but are used as foundations to build on. The device fits 'somewhere'; this and its history make care practices inert and resistant to change rather than prone to revolution.[23]

Articulating positions

What is crucial, then, is the articulation of the shape of the innovative practice. The uncontrolled field study does this by asking what practices the participants created and what they learned from them. What were the aims and what are they now? Did different practices emerge than was expected, promised or hoped for? For instance, what are the implications of replacing professional control with self-management? What works, what does not, and why?

The next question is *who* should articulate all this. Modern researchers engaging patients in medical research as well as researchers conducting disability studies suggest that patients and nurses should be the researchers of their own practices. They can explicate the knowledge they have gained as well as the knowledge embedded in their practices and devices. There are, however, good reasons for inviting others to help them do this. First, very practical: caring and conducting research are entirely different tasks with different aims, each demanding time and specialist skill. I have shown some of the problems of combining care and research, such as the extra workload for nurses, and at worst, conducting bad research while giving suboptimal care. It would be wasteful to make good carers spend time on research. Patients may be just too ill to permit this. On the other hand, uncontrolled field studies are much closer to the nurses' and patients' own practical knowledge and may be more fun to do than administrative tasks or filling in questionnaires.

A more fundamental problem is that much of the participants' knowledge is embodied and tacit, embedded in routines and devices, which makes *observation* from a third-person perspective necessary to articulate it. People are not always consciously aware of routines that have already proven their value or changed tacitly. The technology may have quietly changed the definition of a problem by a change in routine. Difficult situations or shy patients may have urged participants to change plans. In addition, people may not always be in a condition that allows them to give accounts of their own practices.

Uncontrolled field studies involve participants in two ways: as the creative innovators described above and as *positions* – the (good) patient and the (good) nurse – in the practice under scrutiny. It is not merely their *opinion* or *preferences* the uncontrolled field study is after (this would fit the consumer patient described in chapter 5) but also the way they enact the position of being a nurse or a patient in the different con-figurations of devices, carers, patients and others.[24] It is not a contrast between 'interest groups' but an articulation of the practices and inter-dependent positions of nurses, patients, devices and others. Active nurses fitted specialised devices and passive patients; active patients fitted other active patients and more modest devices, and so on. Actual participants need not be physically present in the discussions on their practices, but the research should represent *their positions* in order to reflect upon their desirability.[25] Because carers and cared for have to live and work with the devices, their positions are crucial. Their positions stand for possibilities of what care could look like and for possible ways of living with chronic disease.

The status of articulations: comparisons and involving others

The articulations in the uncontrolled field study consist of the descrip-tion of possibilities for caring, the knowledge and values embedded in care practices and the position of participants. Should everyone take these articulations at face value and automatically accept the 'good' en-acted by a practice? Should everyone assume the truth of practical knowl-edge or celebrate invented positions?

No. The uncontrolled field study then goes on to *question the findings* – first, by *comparing* innovative practices and the knowledge developed in them. Uncontrolled field studies are, preferably, multi-site ethnogra-phies of innovative practices. The comparisons show alternatives and variations. They show the complexities of having people with different diseases and devices, having the same disease in different stages, having different disease combinations, or different uses of the same devices. Different practices all define problems and ways to deal with them dif-ferently. An example is the comparison of the monitoring device and the webcam in chapter 4.

Bringing in *even more* variables, understanding and contrasting alternative outcomes, makes the relevant issues easier to discern. The happiness and security that patients felt because they knew professionals closely monitored them deserve serious analysis, but these values may be related to other values and practices in care such as the webcam practice that gave patients the means to support each other. The uncontrolled field study compares the various positions of nurses, patients, devices and diseases to help in weighing and arguing which practices fit whom best.

The uncontrolled field study then feeds the findings of the participants and the comparisons back into innovative practices but also into *broader debates* on innovation in care. This is a second way of questioning findings, and this works best after the comparisons. Reports on the proceedings of innovations could feed the discussion on telecare ethics and efficiency. The debate could substantiate promises and speculations by reflecting on the intricacies of actual care *events* and the interpretation of these events. How should we understand the results of the uncontrolled field study? Is care developed in innovative practices *good*, and if so, is it preferable to other types of goodness? Is it workable, liveable and affordable? How does the telecare intervention relate to the practical knowledge and normative sensitivities of the practice, and does it develop and strengthen them? How does technological innovation *improve* care practice, for whom and at what cost, and how does one improvement relate to other ways of improving practice?

These matters concern others not directly involved in the innovative practices studied: potential patients, carers, families, caring politicians, industries, and so on. The shaping of health care is a matter of public concern, precisely because it deals with the organisation of patients' lives and the lives of those around them. I bet that *you*, the reader, will have a lot to say about telecare after reading this book. Your reflections, along with those of all concerned others, should also be welcome.

The status of practical knowledge

The practical knowledge and normativities articulated by uncontrolled field studies are suggestions and possibilities for discussion rather than directives or probabilities. They are local rather than universal facts, food for thought rather than final conclusions. As a form of knowledge, uncontrolled field studies relate closely to the practical knowledge applied in the field, not taking it for granted but opening it up to argument and debate, hence improving it. Researchers and field parties need not be *trusted* but should encourage debate and welcome *disagreement* on what health care could or should be.

The big difference with classic research methods is that uncontrolled field studies do not keep the kitchen doors closed but instead wide open to involve witnesses to promote collective learning. Researchers are independent of the participants and organisations involved in the innovation, or at least some of the researchers should be.[26] They are independent yet must be *involved* in care practices. They should relinquish rigid surveys and fixed variables to observe the unpredictable outcomes enacted and explicated by the practices in action. In an uncontrolled field study, researchers need to ask open questions and be interested in the intricacies and specificities of the innovative care practices and those living them. They have to assess the possibilities and problems of very different care practices carefully. Instead of sticking to 'pure' methods and rigid designs, researchers need to adapt their methods to make their field inform them. Researchers should articulate and add to the practical knowledge of their field, employing *know-now* strategies, comparative analysis and discussion.

This set-up does not fit the demands of a market where knowledge is a closely guarded good exploited only to stay ahead of the competition. Making innovators keep the doors open to allow collective learning may well be a task for a cautious government that does not want to impose too many decisions on the field. At least it would allow the field and citizens to become interested and involved, to learn from and reflect on local experiences. The telecare industry might also see the sense of opening doors and pursuing shared goals: as it is now, telecare is still a risky business.

Discussions unleashed by an uncontrolled field study

By way of illustration, here is the researcher's view of several themes that emerged from the case studies and warrant discussion. What did the study of these practices show?

Promises, practices and close patients

On the soapbox, telecare promised more efficient use of human resources and/or cost reduction in care. It promised improved quality by helping patients engage in self-management. This would enhance efficiency, support the patients' own wish to be actively involved in their own care, and help keep them living at home rather than in an institution. Professionals could become less active, which would allow for efficient management of staff shortage, or they could become more active to prevent crises and induce security in patients. The normative *threat* was that implementing cold technology would make care devoid of human contact.

The experimental practices showed that care at a distance is often *more intense* than otherwise because contact between patients and carers becomes more frequent. Professionals often initiated the frequent contact,

INNOVATING CARE INNOVATION

particularly when monitoring symptoms. Patients contacted each other more frequently as well in order to exchange practical knowledge.

There is much to say in favour of care at a distance that intensifies contact between patients: it implies interesting roles for people with chronic diseases without making them so dependent on professional care that they have to stay at home to get the care they want. This type of care also takes seriously the need for social contact and the hazards of loneliness, particularly in old age.[27] I would expect this type of care to be helpful and relatively cheap. Befriended patients are great 'low-threshold' carers for their peers, and their friendship and shared needs provide reciprocal relations and continuity in care as well as advice for daily life problems, advice that professional carers do not always provide. The investment required would be for equipment and organisation of patients, demanding a rather more coaching and initiating role for professional carers. The potential of patients to become each others' carers may lead to interesting new social roles, such as becoming *professional* carers trained in using their experiential knowledge.[28]

But there are problems as well. It is hard to fit innovative systems of patients caring for patients into the current system of health care funding in the Netherlands, between central care funding through health insurance companies and the government versus social welfare funding through local municipalities. Chronic patients coaching other chronic patients as a *health care practice* does not fit this two-tiered organisation, although there are local exceptions (often funded by health care organisations). However, the situation may change if health insurers see the effect of improvements in quality of care and efficiency reflected by a reduced demand for the services of professional carers.

This form of care is in an especially fresh experimental phase. The flourishing community of caring patients in this book arose from embedding webcams in practices where patients knew each other intimately. This allowed patients to decide whom they wanted to stay in touch with. To organise *new* caring communities among people who do not know each other demands creativity, as the homecare organisation's webcam experiment showed. As an alternative, care for people with chronic diseases could be organised partly in groups, for instance in general practices. Uncontrolled field studies could follow up on the results.

Close professionals

There are situations where more intense professional care might be legitimate, such as in the practice of palliative care for the oncology patients. The telecare system fits the situation of patients who suffer in silence instead of turning to the doctor for timely treatment. It also fits the aims of this practice: patients are not trained to become self-managers but need instead to come to terms with their changed prospects in life and their imminent death. The professionals take care of symptoms or side effects. The participants achieved the goals of this practice without criticism, bar solving the problem of who cares for the administration of the system or the research.

For the COPD and heart failure patients, this was different. It seems that intensified professional control could keep patients out of the hospital, at least for a while. Yet there were worries, too: about the desirability of professional surveillance, the sense and feasibility of daily measurements, the relation between telecare and other forms of self-care and the reduced responsibility of the patients. Increased control by professionals would give patients no other opportunities to develop their practical knowledge, whereas their condition demands that they do this anyway. Telecare devices cannot take disease away. They do not cook or carry people from one place to another. For people with COPD or heart failure, it is never an option to 'leave it all to the professionals' or to their devices.

To place 'care for symptoms' in the foreground, as happened in the monitoring practices, runs the risk of framing only *one* version of problems as the most relevant, and this may frustrate the capacity for self-care that patients have to engage in anyway. The daily battles with salt-free diet and reduced fluid intake melted into the background in the version of the trouble defined by the monitoring devices, even when it was still central to patients. For the COPD patients, crises were also relevant, and they found it particularly hard to decide when to go to the doctor or take medication. Yet their daily worries were about how to keep moving and do meaningful things when short of breath. These problems have a huge impact on daily life, even though they may fall outside narrow medical definitions of treatment.

Close technologies

Whatever type of (tele)care analysed, 'self-management' turned out to be a misleading term. There was always some form of 'together management', even if the caring partners varied at times. They could be professional carers, telecare devices or fellow patients. Family members, where present, were always involved in one way or another. Rather than understanding care as a practice for treating individuals, it makes sense to look at care in its various configurations, including the place of technology and the relations made with and through it. This gives a better idea of which configurations are worth arguing for or against.

Close research

Uncontrolled field studies fit innovative care practices where not much knowledge is at hand and where the stakes are high. These studies use and develop the practical knowledge of participants in the innovative practices. It shows how practices shape problems, how participants deal with them and why this would be good. Uncontrolled field studies help to reflect upon normative matters that are not imaginary but actually emerge in practice. A well-known complaint about conventional research is that its outcomes are clear but nobody knows what they mean or what to do with them. Classic research is far too remote from the practices it studies to provide the answers to the thorny questions of how to understand innovations. Uncontrolled field studies are not. Results of uncontrolled field studies are directly relevant to the question of whether and which telecare devices improve care practices, even if they provide no simple answer. Uncontrolled field studies support the improvement of care practices rather than prove the effectiveness of machines.[29]

Fitting research does not harm the object of research in the widest sense of the term 'harm'. Scientific research may damage the organisation of innovative practices or even damage care when research methods are blind to its important characteristics. The knowledge created in uncontrolled field studies is analytic and traceable; it explicates how it names and frames its object. The ethics of scientific research does not define the conditions for research but forms the core of conducting research. Research that fits is *caring* research; it can be used to improve the practices it studies. Ironically, the *efficiency* gains of uncontrolled field studies concern the better organisation of *research* practices. Telecare innovation is managing to take place against the odds, but so far there is an abundance of evaluation that fits neither the requirements of classic evaluation research nor the innovative care practices. Employing flexibly designed uncontrolled field studies could prevent these misfits.

However, after finishing this book, even the least suspicious reader will no longer take promises or changes in routines at face value. It is high time to organise some uncontrolled field studies and study their workings – in uncontrolled field studies.

Acknowledgements

There are many people to thank for their help with the research and the writing of this book. It has been said before: doing research is a collective effort. To acknowledge this, I have written these notes of thanks in the shape of movie credits. The credits mean to say 'thank you' but instead show what everybody has contributed so that the reader can be properly impressed.

The cast

It is good custom to start with the cast, the people who move around on the pages. I cannot name them, because I guaranteed them anonymity. The stars 'act naturally' in this book that is not a work of fiction. The book is also not a mere reportage, because of the structuring work of the concepts and comparisons, and the choices I made about what to tell and how to tell it. But it *is* documentary in the sense that this book is about real people, real concerns and real practices. The book makes use of the practical knowledge and normative findings of the informants, the people who have lived and worked with the telecare technologies. In this sense, this book is a true co-production, telling a story that none of us could have told separately. For this, I cannot thank them enough.

The crew

Executive production
The research started in 2005 with a grant from NWO, The Netherlands Organisation for Scientific Research, from the Ethics, Research and Policy programme: Care at a distance. A normative investigation into telecare. The book was written during the EFORTT research programme funded by the European Community's seventh Framework programme: Ethical Frameworks for Telecare Technologies for older people at home.

Production manager
Margo Trappenburg, editor of the Care and Welfare series
Without Margo, this book would never have been written.

Location management, props and grips
AMC, department of General Practice, Section of Medical Ethics

Proofreaders and focus pullers
Amade M'charek, Annemarie Mol, Jan Pols and Dick Willems

Indispensable for the first draft of a manuscript ('done!') are the proof-readers ('... but not yet...'). Amade seems to always know what I am trying to get at, even in my most premature philosophical gropings; she always helps me to articulate my thoughts better – and isn't that what thinking is all about! Amade also gave me the idea for the final framing of the book and celebrated the 'birth of the manuscript' with me. Anne-marie, leaving her eating bodies for a while, chewed on many little flaws in the text and urged me to re-write it to make it easier to swallow and digest for the reader. She seasoned her comments by adding a hand of little '+++' sometimes with a delicious added '!' These gave the revision of the manuscript real zest. Jan proudly volunteered as 'the educated lay reader', pointing out incomprehensible sections, sloppy arguments and places where diplomacy might just be more suitable than irony. I think that is quite something for a dad! Dick has a very specific way of commenting on drafts; there are not many notes, but those that are there truly lift one's thinking to a higher level. I hope there will be many texts and crucial notes to follow!

Advice, support, colleagues and co-researchers
* My colleagues from the NWO project:
Maartje Schermer and Corrette Ploem

I will never forget how Maartje and I went for our first interview in this field that was new to us. Nobody answered the door, the telecare company seemed to have disappeared. We later learnt that it had gone bankrupt, a phenomenon that turned out not to be uncommon in this field. It was great to do interviews together in projects that *did* survive.

* The advisory board
Daan Dohmen, Sjef Gevers, Arie Hasman, Medard Hilhorst, Annemarie van Hout, Ellen Maat, Jan Thie and Jelle van der Weijde

After this bewildering start, we were supported by an advisory board that helped us understand what was going on and suggested new angles and visions.

* My colleagues from the EFORTT (EC) project
From Lancaster University: Maggie Mort, Christine Milligan and Celia Roberts
From the Autonomous University in Barcelona: Blanca Callén, Miquel Domenèch, Daniël López, Thomás Sánchez-Criado, Francisco Tirado
From the Diakonhjemmet in Oslo: Ingunn Moser and Hilde Thygesen

I warmly recommend a European project to any researcher. Not only are the local differences extremely enriching for the research, they also learn much about habits of diet and sports. Imagine dinner at 11.00 pm in Barcelona, with the slight wind still warm and the wine seductively red... Potato chips are essential for lunch in England, preferably in Lancaster's Butterfly House or while chewing on the thoughts of Emanuel

Swedenborg in his beautiful former residence in London. And imagine Nordic skiing and sleighing in the all-white mountains of Norway! I really enjoyed our sessions together and I hope we will find ways to continue our research (and outings!) in the future.

* My colleagues from the AMC's philosophy of care
Annemarie van Hout, Antje Seeber , Beate Giebner, Ben de Bock, Erik Olsman, Esther Leuthold, Jean Philipe de Jong, Mirjam Broerse, Myra van Zwieten, Sabine Ootes, Susanne de Kort, Trudie Gerrits and Yolande Witman
It is great to be infected by your enthusiasm and it is a privilege to work together with some of you closely.

* My colleague in all of the above
Dick Willems
Dick is the manager of the Section of Medical Ethics, with its atmosphere of possibility and trying out new ideas – ideas that seem to suit *him* quite naturally. Dick has been essential for the course my work has taken. He is great fun to be with and a tremendously generous reader of drafts. I look forward to our explorations of the aesthetics of daily life and care!

Interviewer
Ether Leuthold
Esther patiently interviewed telecare users of the PAL4 project as well as project leaders for the EFORTT study. It was great working together with Esther as a sparring partner and wonderful to have her as a companion in fieldwork – and in walks during lunchhour.

Intellectual support, Dutch summers, jamu and skype
Hans Pols

Script editor
Ragini Werner, Needser (Native English Editing Service)
'Spring cleaning' was the word that came to my mind when I got the manuscript back from Ragini; I am sure she would have picked a better word!

Cover photography and visual effects
Ruud Mast
Life is barren without art. Ruud makes life more beautiful.

Artefact and aartivark philosophy
Auke Pols

True love, sine-qua-nons, grounding, fun, travel and animals
Bertus Eskes
Flo

Very special thanks
Ingunn Moser
For providing ever more pieces of the expanding jigsaw of our research
with work, comments and friendship.

Amade M'charek
Institutional academic life may sometimes feel like swimming against
the tide. However, any fatigue instantly changes into inspiration and
flow during the theoretical explorations, the sharing of fascinations and
the 'pushing of concepts' with wonderful Amade. The combination of
friendship and intellectual work moves me more than I can say.

Inspirational thought sharing
Vicky Singleton, Henriette Langstrup, Brit Ross Winthereik, Hans Harbers, Myriam Winance, Kristin Asdal, Estrid Sörensen, Thomas Schef-
fer, Wilma Boevink, Rosemarie Buikema, Dorine Bauduin, Antoinette
de Bont, Iris Wallenburg, Jolanda Habraken, Jacqueline Kool, Detlef
Petry, Carolien Smits, Evelien Tonkens, John Law, Jannelle Taylor,
Geertje Boschma, Ant Lettinga, Rob Hagendijk, Maureen McNeil, Car-
men Romero Bachiller, Marjo Rauhalla, Sjaak van der Geest, Ingrid
Baart

Continuing on-line support
HanneLore Modderkolk

Dinners
Robert Jan Both, Irma Roose, Marja Depla, Jet Isarin, Karen Wegner

Appendix: Projects studied for this book

1   Oncology & COPD patients

Telecare practice	Palliative care for people with cancer	Homecare for people with COPD/long-term illnesses	Rehabilitation clinic for COPD & asthma
Project/permanent	Project	Permanent, but pending financial arrangements	Permanent
Type of device	Health Buddy	Health Buddy/white box (for COPD only), webcam, touch screen and computer	Webcam and computer
Period of use by patients/implemented?	3 months/no	Permanent	3 months/yes
Fieldwork	16 home visits; Interviews with 14 patients, including 6 with partner 1 widow 1 specialist nurse: several times; Project group meetings	13 home visits & interviews with patients; Interviews with 4 nurses, the general project manager (several times), 2 local project managers	6 months in clinic; Interviews with 9 patients at home; 2 volunteers; 2 central carers; 2 technicians, 1 manager; 1 project manager; Project coordinator: several times
Organisation	General hospital	3 home care organisations	National clinic
Demographics	North NL	Middle & South NL	Central NL
Patients involved	64 (58 in control condition retrospectively)	No information (projects in starting phase)	About 20 in any given period
Professionals involved	4 oncology nurses	COPD nurses	social workers

2 Cardiac patients

Telecare practice	Care for people with heart failure	Care for people with heart failure
Project/permanent	Project, longstanding	Project
Type of device	Health Buddy/white box	Monitoring blood pressure, weight, pulse. Informative videos. Call centre.
Period of use by patients/implemented?	3 months/longstanding use, ever new research	Permanent/stopped in most hospitals after RCT
Fieldwork	Interviews: 1 heart failure nurse 3 patients 2 telephone interviews with producers of device	Interviews: 3 heart failure nurses 5 patients visiting the hospital 1 representative of industry 1 cardiologist 1 interview with call centre staff: doctor, nurse, coordinator. 1 technician installing devices at home Observation of work of call centre nurse. 2 home visits to patients
Organisation	Hospital	5 hospitals, 1 studied. Call centre
Demographics	South NL	All over NL
Patients involved	66	98 (113 in control condition)
Professionals involved	4 heart failure nurses, 1 cardiologist	Many heart failure nurses, cardiologists

3   Projects studied in less detail

Telecare practice	Webcam project in homecare, east NL	Webcam project homecare and hospital	Diabetes care general practice and hospital
Project/permanent	No information after bankruptcy of organisation	Project	Project
Type of device	Webcam	Webcam	Health Buddy/white box
Period of use by patients/implemented?	Variable/ yes	Variable/ no	3 months/yes
Fieldwork	Interview with project coordinator	Interview with service organisation, innovation manager, insurance company (funding the project)	Interview with diabetes nurse and project coordinator
Organisation	Homecare		General practice, hospital
Demographics	East NL	North NL	West NL
Patients involved	No information	No information	No information
Professionals involved	Homecare nurses		Internal doctors, diabetes nurses

Other projects
One homecare project went bankrupt before we could interview staff (hence not listed in table). Two homecare projects failed when homecare organisations went bankrupt.

Conferences and meetings
We attended conferences as well as demonstrations and presentations by the industry, e-health presentations from national patient organisations, and so on. We studied project documentation and followed public discussions.

Citizen panels
We organised five panels for the EU study, three in 2008, two in 2010. We invited telecare users, potential users and people caring for their elders to discuss their views on telecare developments.

The first three panels discussed the participants' notions of good care and problems they feared or wanted to see solved. We introduced tele-care technology in the second part of the meeting: a monitoring device for heart failure; webcam communication with a professional carer or informal carer; internet & email; alarms & sensors; robot pets.

We organised a meeting to discuss preliminary findings from the ethnographic studies. Also, the findings from the first round of citizen panels was fed back to participants, and some results from other countries were also presented.

EU partners
Ethnographic material, analyses and papers from the European partners participating in the European study were also used as a background for the Dutch case studies. Participating countries were Great Britain, Spain and Norway.

Notes

Notes Chapter 1

1. See Currell et al. 2000.
2. Examples of 'old' telecare technology, in use for some time in the Netherlands but not part of the hype (this differs from country to country) include thrombosis monitoring at a distance and the use of personal alarms. These are both quite 'normalised', as Carl May and colleagues (2007) would put it, meaning that the technology is routinely embedded and taken for granted in everyday practice.
3. For the dreams of the national Dutch health care consumer organisation, see Tjalsma 2007.
4. In the Netherlands, telecare did not promise that patients would have better *access* to health care services, as was the case with the first developments in telemedicine in countries like Canada and the US (see Mort, May & Williams 2003). Cartwright (2000) gives a fascinating critical analysis of the politics of telemedicine, where vulnerable poor populations are used to test technology for the army and space travel. She also points to the hegemony of dominant medical centres over local knowledge and health care practices. For this argument, see also Miscione 2007. For examples of telemedicine in remote places in Canada, see Roberge et al. 1982 and Dunn et al. 1980. For critical notes on utopian thinking by decision makers see Berg 2002.
5. See Onor & Misan 2005; Sparrow 2002; Sparrow & Sparrow 2006 for some vivid nightmares, and for an overview of nightmarish positions: Pols & Moser 2009.
6. The 'sociology of expectations' is a branch of STS concerned with the way the sciences generate hope – and money – besides facts. It shows that public promises in the short term always overrate the practical possibilities of technology, whereas in the long term they are usually completely wrong. The behaviour of technology users seems very hard to predict, and large sums of money may turn out to have been wasted. See Brown 2003; Brown & Michael 2003; Borup et al. 2006.
7. Interestingly, notions of what telecare promises to do, what the exact problem of an aging population is and how telecare would help to solve the problems differs greatly across EU countries. For instance, the Netherlands is targeting telecare solutions at elderly people with chronic diseases, whereas in Spain and England the target group is the general aging population. The concern is that the elderly will live alone, away from their children. The ways in which the actors take telecare promises seriously also differs: the Dutch government is positive, but leaves it to 'the field' and the market to develop telecare solutions; the English NHS is actively implementing telecare in the homes of older people. See for the UK situation: May, Finch, Mair & Mort 2005; Milligan, Mort & Roberts 2010; Milligan Roberts & Mort 2010. For Spain: López 2010 and Norway: Thygesen & Moser (2010). Schillmaier and Domènech (2010) collects most of these papers.
8. See Barbot 2006 for different types of 'active patients'.

9. More about the promises in Chapters 4, 6 & 7. Promises are typical in policy literature and in communications from the industry. In the Netherlands a recent report from the board advising the government on matters of health care organisation (Raad voor de Volksgezondheid en Zorg, RVZ, 2010), has put reasoning about telecare and more efficient use of working capacity firmly on the health care policy agenda.

10. More about the nightmares in Chapters 2 & 3. The literature on the *ethics* of technology often hosts the nightmares, see note 4.

11. See www.euractiv.com/en/health/doctors-unconvinced-ehealth-policy/article-170213, published 8 February 2008, last accessed 22 August 2010.

12. López & Domènech (2009) beautifully analyse how wearing pendant alarms (necklace holding a personal alarm button) evokes an ambivalent identity of being both *vulnerable* (one runs the risk of falling and needing help at any time, even in the space always thought of as safe: the home) and, more heroically, *autonomous*, capable of living independently at home. López describes how these personal alarms must try to optimise and combine the effect of each of these identities on health and well-being (López 2010). See Thygesen (2009) for an analysis of the workings of smart home technology in sheltered housing for people with dementia.

13. This is very different from the situation in Great Britain, where the NHS actively directs telecare development by setting targets for the implementation of telecare projects (see Milligan, Roberts & Mort 2010; Roberts, Mort & Milligan 2010). The Dutch health care market is not a 'free' market, but the government defines the conditions under which it allows it to work.

14. Trappenburg (2008) and Van de Bovenkamp & Trappenburg (2010) show that the national patient organisation (NPCF) is organised and financed by the government, who needed the patients as a party (the consumers) on the health care market to be constructed. Hence, the organisation is less about representing patients and their concerns, and more about the desire to create health care as a market with critical consumers who want value for money. This may explain why this organisation took sides in the telecare debate so quickly.

15. A concern in offering telecare devices to patients that studies rarely address is what it means if telecare organisations take devices away after a pilot or pre-fixed time slot. Many projects in this study started to offer telecare for a restricted period, but many patients (and so far: successfully) objected to their device being taken away at the appointed date. The setting of a period of use often had an economic background but has great implications for patients.

16. See Finch et al. 2003.

17. The 1950s saw the design of quantitative studies, within the paradigm of evidence-based medicine since the 1980s, with the randomised controlled trial (RCT) as the gold standard of good research. See for example Sehon & Stanley (2003) for an explanation, or Timmermans and Berg 2003 for a study of the rise of evidence-based medicine. The pharmaceutical industry became legally obliged to use RCTs before they could think of marketing new drugs: RCTs should prove them effective.

18. Eminoviç et al. 2007 complain about this in the context of telemedicine projects they have been evaluating in a meta-analysis, an aggregation of trial results.

19. There is some useful literature with comparable demonstrations about the use of standards in care (Berg 1997; Timmermans, Bowker & Star 1998). These authors stress that systems and standards do indeed change health care practice but that the effects differ greatly because people using them negotiate and change the standards when they use them. How protocols work out is hard to predict; it needs empirical and local studies to show what their effects are, before their acceptability can be discussed (Mol & Berg 1998).

20. See Pols & Willems (2011) for this argument. John Law (1994) uses the term 'projectness' for conceptions of interventions as discrete events, with a clear beginning and ending and a linear way of discerning cause and effect.

21. See Lettinga 2000; Lettinga & Mol 1999. The word 'effect' is somewhat misleading here because, strictly speaking, there is no linearity where a cause produces an effect that one may consequently identify. See also chapter 8.

22. Scholars often make the same argument about pharmaceutical industries. See, for example, Healey 2002. The debate in the Netherlands about these kind of issues was stirred up after the publication of a book by Dehue (2008) evoking heated debates involving many angry psychiatrists.

23. The short history of telecare shows the frequent collapse of telecare projects after a project has finished. See Langstrup-Nielsen 2005; Finch et al. 2003. See Mort, May & Williams (2003) for different ways in which RCTs and their ending interfered with dermatology telemedicine practices.

24. The term articulation is from Dona Haraway (1991) and signifies that stories, scientific analyses or other articulations are never 'neutral' but always specific, highlighting some matters rather than others. I take it as the normative contribution of researchers to consider carefully why they use these concepts rather than others. This normativity is about sensitivity for concepts. See Pols 2008 and the final chapter of this book.

25. Wittgenstein's parallel to the 'language game' may be instructive here. According to Wittgenstein, a word does not merely refer to an 'object out there' but to other words within a particular language game. The language game is the order that produces the specific meaning of a term rather than its dictionary meaning. See e.g. Wittgenstein 1953.

26. That objects may have 'versions' points to a notion of 'multiplicity' that is part of the naming and framing theories informing this study. The exemplary work here is Annemarie Mol (2002). Multiplicity of objects means that people enact objects in different ways within different practices. As Mol shows, atherosclerosis is a different object in epidemiology, pathology or the clinic. This is not a matter of different *interpretations* of the object but of *ontological* differences: the object *is* different things in different practices. See also: Law & Mol 2007. See Moreira (2006) for different 'blood-pressures'.

27. For empirical analyses of how ideals of good care are embedded in practices and technology, see Thygesen & Moser 2010; Mol 2010; Willems 2010, 2003; Pols 2008. Different from an ethics of care, where ethicists mostly define care as inherently good or a normative framework for good care is developed (Joan Tronto 1993 is the exemplary philosopher here), an analysis of care practices may show that well-intended activities may turn out to be undesirable practices. Such analyses are attentive to care practices' *orienta-*

tion towards doing good but make the *result* of this orientation the object of empirical study.

28. To think about the normative sides of these modes of ordering, I have been inspired by Boltanski and Thévenot (1991). Boltanski and Thévenot framed a theoretical vocabulary that allows one to study how ordinary people justify their actions. They discerned different 'repertoires of justification'. People draw upon these repertoires in varied ways, using different types of justification in the same situation. Nevertheless, each repertoire, in and of itself, is internally consistent and has its own hierarchy of values and its own conception of the world.

29. There is a parallel to Wittgenstein's language games, explicitly including material objects in them. Michel Foucault and Georges Canguilhem also inspire my particular position, where the *object* brought into being in knowledge practices is analysed as a position within particular relations. I draw upon studies in ANT using the notion of 'enactment', see e.g. Mol 1998; 2002. The best description of material semiotics is given by John Law, where he describes the need to study reality as it takes shape within 'material semiotic networks'. In a material semiotic network, 'entities take their form and acquire their attributes as a result of their relations to other entities' (Law 1999, p. 3). 'Things' and humans are not something solid in and of themselves, but their identities come into being within their local connections to other things and humans.

30. See Pols & Willems 2011. We were building on the work on domestication theory of Lie & Sørensen 1996; Silverstone 2005; Silverstone et al. 1992; Berker et al. 2006. However, see also Webster (2002) and Callén et al. (2009) for a discussion that Health Technology assessment involving deliberations on the design process with (potential) users is not enough to capture the creative engagements of users who subvert, appropriate, refuse or adopt new technology. See Anestad (2003) for an analysis of what she calls 'design of configurations', this being the creation of a well-working mix of people, practices and artefacts, a process in which the introduced technology produces changes and is also changed itself. For the domestication of animals and plants, see Haraway 2008 and Clutton-Brock 1998.

31. Studies reflecting on material semiotics use other terms as well: ANT, after-ANT (see Gad & Bruun Jensen 2010), empirical philosophy (Mol 2000) and praxiography (Mol 2002). This re-naming serves the freedom to build on as well as subvert and re-invent a theoretical 'tradition' that aims to constantly innovate its own terms and conditions. Scholars argue for this with more or even more irony: see, for example, Pickering 1992; Law 1997; Latour 1991.

32. See e.g. Lichtenstein 2010.

33. See Fisher 1992.

34. The example is from Bruno Latour 1999. See Verbeek 2009 for ethical considerations on persuasive technology.

35. Foucault 1971.

Notes Chapter 2

1. See Habermas 1985. See Mol (2008) for a critique of distinguishing 'care' as a space next to other spaces.
2. This is common in an ethics of care, with Joan Tronto (1993) as the exemplary philosopher. Ethicists of care often pursue universal definitions. See Pols 2006 and Brown 2010 for an empirical approach to what care and goodness are in particular situations.
3. Foucault 1973; Osborne 1992; Struhkamp et al. 2008.
4. The development of the power/ knowledge metaphor seems to derive from a mix of 'Birth of the clinic' (1973) and 'Discipline and punish' (1977).
5. See Pols & Moser 2009 for a critical discussion.
6. See e.g. Ihde 1991 for an image of a non-technological utopia. Although it is difficult to take his image of pristine beaches seriously, the underlying fear of alienation is present in many discussions about the social effects of internet use.
7. Telecare devices form a strange set of devices here. They are not medical technologies because they are brought in from outside medical practice. Yet they can only function within medical practices and, to that end, need to become medical devices.
8. Dick Willems (2010) shows a case where a family considered a dead person's spectacles acceptable technology for him to wear in the coffin, whereas nasal cannula were removed even though the deceased used to wear them daily. Apparently, boundaries of which technology 'belongs' to us shift.
9. The assumed functionality of medical technology is also an example of the idea that technology *determines* what will happen when people start using it. See, for instance, Wyatt 2008. Interestingly, both the promises and nightmares of telecare development assume that technology is the determining factor, see Chapter 1.
10. See Mol 2008 for the way in which industries design blood sugar measuring devices to target different user groups.
11. Sparrow & Sparrow 2006; 2002; Gamon et al. 1998.
12. This is a widespread fear: it was prominent in the citizens' panels we organised to discuss telecare in care with (potential) elderly users; see also: Milligan, Mort & Roberts, 2010. Roberts & Mort (2009) and Oudshoorn (2009) point to the tendency of telecare technology (and discourses on this technology) to fragment care and favour reductionist images of 'telepatients' (Mort, Finch & May 2009). The more subjective aspects in care may be threatened or may become separated from 'hands-on' care work.
13. There have been many discussions on the socialising versus the de-socialising effects of the internet and other new media. In the Netherlands, even the queen interfered in this debate in her 2009 Christmas speech by warning of the superficiality of electronic contacts. This sparked off much debate in the newspapers.
14. A fifth argument that Sparrow & Sparrow address does not return in this paper: this is the objection of having oneself or others (like frail elderly) be *cheated* by thinking that machines do things they are not capable of, such as loving their owners. Instead of judging deception beforehand, however, in this chapter I will look at the perceptions expressed by those participating in these practices, and cheating was not among them.

15. Unpredictability may, however, be programmed, as AIBO the robot dog shows. This indeed makes it much more interesting than devices with a high degree of predictability, creating a good fit as a companion. See Pols & Moser 2009.

16. Implicitly, this seems to imply that a 'willingness to sacrifice something' is a test to see if a relation is caring or not: only a friend in need is a friend indeed. One could, however, also argue that it may be valuable to be engaged in less demanding relations, such as with robot dogs that may be loved but do not urinate on the carpet or need to be walked (see Pols & Moser 2009).

17. There is some dispute about the meaning of the term 'palliative care'. On the one hand, it seems to refer to 'a kind of care' where 'quality of life' rather than a 'cure' is the goal. As such, palliative care seems to best fit cancer patients; professionals worry about comfort and pain, and the patient does not have to be active in care but has to come to terms with the end of life. Other patients, like COPD and heart failure patients, cannot be that passive in their own care. They will have to take care of themselves until they die, as professionals cannot take over. The idea of palliative care as a kind of care seems to be behind the palliative care programme of the Dutch financer of health research, ZonMw (swww.zonmw.nl/nl/onderwerpen/alle-program-ma-s/palliatieve-zorg/) when they speak about 'the new care model'. On the other hand, when palliative care is used to denote a particular *phase in care* – i.e., care in the final stages of life – phrases such as 'palliative care should be started earlier' are meaningless. Would this imply that we have to start facing death at an earlier point? Or that quality of care should be the aim of care along with curative aspects? In the latter situation, the opposition between care and cure is unclear. The WHO definition is not conclusive here (WHO 1998).

18. I made 15 home visits. I talked to seven male and seven female patients, including six patients and their partners (three female, three male), and one recent widow.

19. All names in this book are fictitious.

20. The term is from Kleinman & Van der Geest 2009. For studies that take daily life as a starting point, see: Mol 2008; Willems et al. 2006; Winance 2007; Moser 2005 Nijhof 2001; Corbin & Strauss 1988.

21. Of course, *real* art may just do this. The point here is the practical functionality that is part of the aesthetics.

22. For the concept of tinkering, referring to the process of caring by adapting to changing situations, see chapter 5. The notion of fitting brings out the normative or successful moments within this process of tinkering.

23. 64 patients participated in the project (Korsten 2010). The project manager said that 'there weren't many refusers, about five, but those who were there handed their white box back in the first week they had it.' Others [among my informants] stopped when the chemotherapy ended. The project manager told me that so far, they had been very flexible as to how long people could have the device. This had to do with the budget that could afford more patients than were actually included [Minutes of project group meeting, 4 December 2009].

24. Reference to 'too much' care exists elsewhere as well when concerning the independence of patients or the goal of care to make people independent or not make them dependent (see e.g. Pols 2008; Struhkamp et al. 2009).

Although professional carers do not mention independence as an ideal or goal in palliative care, it returns in the shape of care that is 'good enough' – not too little and not in excess.

25. See Suchman 2007; Turkle 1984; Wilson 2005; Haraway 1991.

Notes Chapter 3

1. Part of this analysis is published as Pols 2009.
2. That technology sets norms is also put forward in the idea that technology has a script (Akrich 1992; Latour 1992). As in movies and plays, technology can be seen as containing scripts that direct their users/players as to what characters they are, what they should do when and how to do it well.
3. See Mol 2002; Willems 2003; Pols 2008. The term enactment signifies that the participants are not always aware of the norms they enact. Devices and taken-for-granted routines may tacitly hide these norms.
4. 'Good nursing' is obviously not static or ahistorical; it is related to many local developments, the introduction of new technology, buildings, different types of patients, organisations and changing notions of what is 'good care' and 'good knowledge' in both nursing and other disciplines (Nicolini 2006; Greatbatch et al. 2005; Lehoux et al. 2002; May et al. 2001).
5. The name of the conference was 'Telecare: Dialogue and Debate – The emergence of new technologies and responsibilities for healthcare at home in Europe' and took place in Utrecht, Netherlands, 20-21 September 2007. It is well documented: see http://www.csi.ensmp.fr/WebCSI/MEDUSE/, last accessed: 28 July 2008
6. Van Kammen, 2002; Willems 2004.
7. Norman 2006; Gammon et al. 1998; Sävenstedt al. 2005.
8. Bauer 2004; Onor & Misan 2005; Milligan et al. 2006.
9. Miller 2006; Greatbatch et al. 2005; Smith & Godfrey 2002; Tuckett 2002.
10. In the horror image of the abandoned, technologically mediated patient, *nobody* is looking after the patient. Implicit in the nightmare of coldness is that there are no other people around the patient to provide embodied relations, only the nurse.
11. Maartje Schermer was my fellow researcher on the first telecare project.
12. Personal communication on a presentation by the author at a conference, September 2010.
13. Soon, the idea of preventing crises was linked to notions of cost reduction. There has been a shift in public notions of the benefits of telecare: preventing disease exacerbation will lead to cost reduction in health care because it saves money by not having to admit patients to (expensive) hospitals. These notions only appeared in nursing talk when enthusiastic carers looked for ways to make their telecare practice financially viable. They never trusted that quality of care and patient satisfaction were good enough reasons to have telecare financed by insurance companies or by the government (AWBZ).

Notes Chapter 4

1. This is termed multiplicity when it concerns several problems that go by the same name. See Annemarie Mol (2002) for different enactments of atherosclerosis.

2. 'Enactment' includes activities embedded in devices as well as activities that are possibly outside the conscious awareness of participants. My use of the term highlights another aspect – i.e. that the identity of a patient's problem may come about through the way it is 'done' in relation to activities and routines, devices and talk in particular practices.

3. See Winance 2010 for an elegant analysis of how person and wheelchair work together in a meticulous mutual adaptation. See Ross Winthereik & Langstrup (2010) for an unexpected outcome of the new configurations of patients and carers in the practice of using a web-based patient record.

4. For the argument that self-management technology helps construct a 'self', see Willems 2000.

5. Dutch patients tend to find American patients' expressions too exaggerated and sentimental.

6. Maartje Schermer (2009) argues that an aspect of self-management implying compliance to a medical regime complements an idea of self-management needing *concordance* and collaborative elements. In the latter case, patients can utter their concerns and thus be empowered rather than 'taught'. My analysis proves her point but also complicates it by placing 'medical advice' and 'interventions' on different levels. Home use of medication needs more work by patients than just carrying out measurements for the nurse. See Chapter 5 for an elaboration.

7. Kivits (2004) points out that people looking for health information on the internet – often a prototype for the idea of patient self-management – are actually not ill themselves but look up information for sick relatives or try to make their lifestyles even healthier than they already were.

8. López (discussing personal alarms, 2010) argues that we can understand telecare developments best within a move from a governance regime of disciplining patients towards a regime of security. A disciplining regime moulds an ideal subject, whereas a regime of security deals with possible emerging events, good or bad. My analysis identifies both disciplinary and security moments, but the latter are a very specific kind, depending on the kind of device used. One may live with the risk of weight or blood pressure increase, or with the possibility of chatting to other people. The kind of security regime or the type of risks one expects to have to deal with varies greatly.

9. See Oudshoorn & Pinch (2003) for an analysis of the invisible work of home-care nurses and physicians to help enact the patient as a 'competent diagnostic agent'.

10. Moreira (2004), borrowing the term from Callon & Rabéharisoa, prefers to speak of the 'patient collective' instead of 'the patient'; hence there can be no misunderstanding that 'the patient' is not merely the individual, but is always mediated by things, others, devices, and so on. Moreira demonstrates how, within surgical post-operative practices, the relational dynamics of social and material components may re-institute patients' sense of themselves and re-organise their relationship with the world and other people. The out-

come of this dynamic process is the reorganisation of forms of agency for the patient.

11. The process of caring or tinkering is, in addition to being a normative process, also a creative process. For tinkering, see chapter 5.

Notes Chapter 5

1. The relation between biomedicine and patients has always been ambivalent. On the one hand, there are the growing demands for and great public trust in medical practices and treatment, shown by growing investments in Western health care practices. On the other, there are many measures taken to protect patients and strengthen their position, particularly to protect them from research that may hurt the test persons. These measures include guidelines, codes of conduct and new laws. The critical position stems from the gross abuse of medical practices, especially in research that occurred in the 20th century (see e.g. Lederer 1995), during and after World War II (eugenics programmes, see e.g. Proctor 1988; Weindling 1989), but also after that, for instance the Tuskegee syphilis trials. The Tuskegee study aimed to study the course of syphilis infection in humans. The scientists did not inform the subjects in the study about its real purpose. Treatment was available, but the researchers withheld it from their subjects, leading to certain death for most of them. See Reverby 2000; 2009; Brandt 1978. Today, dubious medical research practices are those that recruit poor people from developing countries as research subjects. See Petryna 2007; 2009; Petryna, Lakoff & Kleinman 2006; Cooley 2001; Benatar 2001.

2. See Barbot 2006 for the different ways in which 'active patients' take shape.

3. Books by doctors who have fallen ill and thus finally understand their patients underline this difference. See e.g. Sacks 1984. Experiential knowledge is then only accessible to sufferers, excluding professionals who may be experts in practical knowledge, such as nurses or physiotherapists.

4. See Callén et al. 2009. In medical anthropology, the distinction between disease and illness, where the disease is the biomedical variant of the illness that patients experience, runs the same risk of turning patients' knowledge into matters of culture or beliefs, needing an explanatory model to understand what is by definition different from a biomedical model. See e.g. Eisenberg 1977; Kleinman 1980; Cohen et al. 1994. For a critical analysis of opposing nature and culture and naturalising the body, see Mol & Law 2004; Suyata 2009; M'charek 2010a,b; Mol 2002. For a critique from the disability studies perspective, see Zola 1991; Hughes & Paterson 1997; Shakespeare 2006; Hughes 2009; Moser 2009; Pols 2010a, d Pols & M'charek 2010a, b.

5. See Prior 2003.

6. See also Akrich 2010.

7. See Whelan (2007) on endometriosis, Arksey (1994) on RSI. Whelan re-introduces the term 'epistemic community' (coined by Haas 1992, see Akrich 2010) to refer to the group of people who orient themselves to a particular kind of knowledge by experience. This knowledge includes the experience of dealing with doctors.

8. The term 'orphan disease' comes from Callon & Rabéharisoa (2003) and their orphan disease is muscular dystrophy. AIDS is another example. When it emerged, patients effectively influenced research practices (Epstein 1996).

9. This is the case in the recovery movement in mental health care (see Mowbray et al. 1998). One debate is, for instance, on the necessity and effects of lifelong use of anti-psychotic medication (see Lehman 2004). Long-term effects of these drugs are unknown, even when psychiatrists prescribe these drugs for a lifetime.

10. Epstein 1995.

11. I simplify here. The term 'research in the wild' comes from Callon & Rabéharisoa (2002; 2003; 2008). See also Callon (1999; 2005). It is, however, ambiguous in their work what the difference between 'research in the wild' – i.e. knowledge from patient groups – and laboratory science is. They need to assume there are differences or there would not be a dynamic between the concerned groups and the scientists. What these differences are, however, is unclear. Are there different contents of knowledge, yet comparable – if primitive – methods? Do researchers in the wild ask different questions, leading to knowledge that is equally valued? Or do they ask the same questions but in different ways and spaces of production?

12. Van de Bovenkamp & Trappenburg (2010) show how patients engaged in guideline development can only participate if they can converse with the medical expert in terms of evidence-based knowledge. Scientists often disqualify the knowledge patients bring to the table. If anything, this shows the need for a better understanding of *what it is* that patients may contribute.

13. See Department of Health 2001. See also Edgar, 2005; Greenhalgh 2009; Barbot 2006; Mol 2008.

14. See Henwood et al. 2003; Hart et al. 2004; Kivits 2004; Lupton 1997.

15. There are different ways of looking for symmetries between medical knowledge and knowledge of lay persons or patients. The classic study of Evans-Pritchard (1937) is an example of a symmetrical treatment of local and global rationalities in a non-medical context where he shows the rationality of the Azandes' ways of dealing with rain and rain dances. In his anthropology study of medical anthropologists studying kuru, Anderson (2008) also creates a symmetry but, maybe even more intriguingly, he shows that whiteman's scientific practices may resemble kuru notions of sorcery and even practices of cannibalism more than the scientists would have realised.

16. For the concept of translation or its precursor 'interessement', see Callon 1985; Law 1987; Latour 1987; Callon & Law 1982. For examples in the context of telecare, see Langstrup (2008).

17. In her important analysis of health care, Deborah Lupton relates consumerism to a self that is a general, Giddensian, late modern 'reflexive project of the self'. In this project, people constantly evaluate the self to maximise entrepreneurially the benefits for the self (see also Nettleton 2004). In my analyses, the types of selves and their 'rationalities' may vary: they may be medical, juridical, liberal, relate to different policy aims or may collude with a medical rationality. I try to be sensitive to the various situated configurations of patients and rationalities.

18. See Van de Bovenkamp, Trappenburg & Grit (2010).

19. For a nuanced discussion on how the ideas of evidence-based medicine and patient centeredness compete to organise clinical practice, and the role that modern technology plays, see May, Rapley et al. 2006; May 2006.

20. An interesting example here is 'complementary medicine', a term hiding the fact that many doctors do not see it as complementary at all but as quackery, or at best as 'placebo'. Health insurances, however, pay for complementary medicine. It is an example of valuing patient preferences or demands more than medical rationality.

21. This explains some of the problems in Dutch mental health care, where patient autonomy is protected by the BOPZ law that allows patients' behaviour that their carers would rate as 'not in their interest', e.g. electing not to take anti-psychotic medication and allowing their condition to deteriorate. A juridical notion of 'the patient's interest' collides with a care notion of this interest. See Pols 2003.

22. Canguilhem 1966.

23. For this distinction, see also Struhkamp et al. 2009; Mol 1998; 2010.

24. There are multiple medical logics or rationalities (see Mol 2002). Scientific knowledge is generated in various genres, e.g., epidemiology, pathology, physiology, genetics, and so on. In Canguilhem terms: there is more than one type of laboratory.

25. Osborne 2002, Barry 1995.

26. There are similarities between the medical scientist and the clinician as well. Both the scientist in the lab and the clinician in the outpatient clinic use implicit and explicit knowledge that is embedded in devices and routines in addition to knowledge that is explicitly articulated in language. Both the scientist and the clinician draw upon different, heterogeneous resources. The scientist may, for instance, use lab values as well as clinical outcomes. The clinician may juggle with parameters such as checking if a patient's wheelchair permits the necessary exercises, and if not, how individual exercises could be changed while fitting the exercise programme in with the patient's effort to keep his job. The biggest difference is that scientists ideally write up the knowledge derived from scientific practices in academic papers that publishers include in databases and make accessible to peers and colleagues. Clinicians articulate clinical knowledge in patient files, case reports and medical education, but this often remains implicit.

27. Tinkering comes from the French term 'bricolage', coined by Lévi-Strauss 1966. See also Prior 2003; Barbot & Dodier 2002; Hester 2005; Mol, Moser & Pols 2010.

28. Mol 2006, Mol & Karayalcin 2008; Moser 2010.

29. The clinical knowledge of professionals is under-studied and needs more articulation to make it transportable for sharing and thus improvement. There is the tradition of writing case reports and transferring clinical knowledge through medical education, but scholars seldom reflect upon clinical experience as a form of knowledge. Exceptions are, for instance, Foucault (1973), Toulmin 1976, Jonssen & Toulmin (1988) and Struhkamp et al. (2009). Evidence-based medicine (EBM) has worsened the status of clinical knowledge. EBM aims to correct the subjective judgements of individual doctors in the clinic. See Chapter 8 for a discussion of this point.

30. The situation is even worse for the practical knowledge of patients. This knowledge is rarely studied. There are, of course, exceptions where daily

practices, including medical practices, are analysed, even though knowledge is not explicitly stressed everywhere: Corbin & Strauss 1988; Hendriks 1998; Nijhof 2001; Winance 2001; 2006; 2007; 2010; Moser 2006; Moser & Law 1999; Struhkamp 2004; Pols 2005; Callon & Rabéharisoa 2004; Willems 1995; Mol 2008; Willems et al. 2006.

31. Polanyi 1966. There are many debates in the literature on the interpretation of tacit knowledge. I do not engage in these debates here directly but articulate my take in following the patients around. See Gourlay 2002; 2006; Henry, 2010; Hunter 1991. Examples of questions include: is tacit knowledge individual or collective, can it be articulated, is it an activity of knowing rather than substantive 'knowledge', and is it accessible to the individual using the tacit knowledge?

32. Willems 1992.

33. The expertise embodied in professional know-how may vary according to disciplines (nurses and GPs may demonstrate inhaler use) and the professional's own experience as a patient or carer of patients.

34. It is important to note that my results are a reduction that relates to the researched context of COPD patients. Other situations and diseases may need other kinds of knowledge; see e.g. the impressive interpretational work that must be done by trauma victims suffering from psychosis (Boevink 2006b).

35. Note that propositions are organised according to certain logics, sets of statements or theories, as became clear in the previous chapter. Propositions fit into scientific disciplines or other orderings.

36. One may or may not make this knowledge explicit.

37. As an educational device, it provides propositions, e.g. 'exercise is good for people with heart failure.'

38. Patients need skills for measuring blood pressure. Embedded notions of underlying disease are propositional.

39. See Charmaz, 2003. 'Sensitising concepts offer ways of seeing, organising, and understanding experience; they are embedded in our disciplinary emphases and perspectival proclivities. Although sensitising concepts may deepen perception, they provide starting points for building analysis, not ending points for evading it. We may use sensitising concepts only as points of departure from which to study the data' (p. 259l). Blumer (1954) coined the term sensitising concept, as opposed to definitive concept. 'A definitive concept refers ... to what is common to a class of objects, by the aid of a clear definition in terms of attributes or fixed bench marks. [...] A sensitising concept lacks such specification of attributes or benchmarks and consequently it does not enable the user to move directly to the instance and its relevant content. Instead, it gives the user a general sense of reference and guidance in approaching empirical instances. Whereas definitive concepts provide prescriptions of what to see, sensitising concepts merely suggest directions along which to look' (p. 7), quoted in Bowen 2006.

40. Suchman 2007.

41. For more on the idea of distributing cognition between heads and instruments, see the classic study of Hutchins 1995. For material ways of organising memory, see Bowker 2006.

42. Annie Cohen-Solal gives a moving example of how *things* remember when she quotes poor demented Sartre wailing about having to quit smoking. This was so hard because, he said, 'objects expect to meet me smoking'.

43. See Pols 2010a for the use of mobility scooters.

44. Habraken et al. (2008) found out that many Dutch COPD patients do not get help with these kinds of daily life questions. They see the pneumonolgist once a year and, when they are lucky, a COPD nurse every four months. It depends on the GP whether he or she will be of assistance here, because the patients usually do not ask for help. GPs may feel they have little to offer, looking at medical solutions that are lacking rather than coaching them in daily life problems.

45. See the previous note.

Notes Chapter 6

1. López and Domènech (2008) argue that *immediacy* and therefore *determinacy* with which the telecare device leads to care delivery (say, instant help the moment people need it) is an element that may distinguish one (tele-) care practice from another. The authors argue that the way telecare devices permit the management of *unexpected* or *undetermined* events (ex-inscription) deserves more analysis, as it is somewhat neglected by the attention to standardisation processes (inscription) discussed in Actor Network Theory to explain immediacy. My question about the *openness* of devices concentrates on the determinacy or openness in the *actions* set in motion rather than the *time* (immediacy) in which help may be organised. The two are obviously related but address different concerns. The telecare devices discussed in this book aim to promote some forms of immediacy, but these are never emergencies needing instantaneous responses. In my comparative perspective, I highlight the way these devices help shape specific forms of care in relation to the way the users put these devices to use, requiring both inscriptions and ex-inscriptions as modes of producing action and 'fit'.

2. Sävenstedt et al. 2004. See also Wakefield et al. 2004. In Pols 2010c I analyse how the metaphor or activity of 'seeing' underlies the discussions on webcams. Seeing can be thought of as 'mirroring nature' (Ihde, Heidegger), but it is also analysed as structured and structuring, following the insights of philosophers as varied as Wittgenstein, Foucault and Haraway. My conclusion here was that 'seeing' (like 'being') does not add much to our understanding of particular situations, because seeing is always embedded in a particular activity that structures what is looked at. There is no natural or pre-theoretical way of seeing.

3. See Johnson 2006; Sluiter 2007.

4. Others describe this too; see e.g. Norman (2006), who reports that the majority of users in telepsychiatry rate videoconferencing as 'almost as good' or 'as good' as face-to-face contacts.

5. The exact percentage of communication that is non-verbal varies according to authors and seems impossible to establish. Onor and Misan (2005) state that only 7% of emotional communication takes place verbally. Let's agree that *lots* of communication is non-verbal.

6. See Pols 2010c for a more detailed description.

7. Sävenstedt et al. (2005) describe this. Non-verbal communication on webcams is thought to be impoverished when compared to face-to-face conversation, but it is enriched when compared to the telephone; see Cukor & Baer 1994; Gammon et al. 1998; Sävenstedt et al. 2005.

8. Gammon et al. (1998) report that users of videoconferencing feel they were 'more prepared and structured'. One respondent also reported that he had to 'keep staring at the screen, so as not to lose contact'.

9. The latter number is from Argyle 1990, quoted in Sävenstedt et al. 2005.

10. They are, of course, far more dictatorial technologies than webcams. See for instance Latour's stories about the speed bump that leaves cars no choice but to slow down or the Aramis subway tunnels that allow low trains to pass but not the higher models the competition uses (Latour 1999; 1996). Maybe the panopticon is the most famous oppressive technology that works partly by the 'subjection' of the people enclosed in it (see Foucault 1977). Technology intervening in complex practices mostly lacks this authority. It helps to shape practices but cannot do this on its own.

11. Gammon et al. (1998) also found that participants stated that 'a working alliance characterised by mutual respect and trust' was a prerequisite to starting a successful psychotherapy supervision relation by webcam (p. 414).

12. For a discussion of the issues of intrusiveness and control, see Fisk 1997; 1998; Milligan, Mort & Roberts 2010.

13. Andrew Barry (1995) argues with Foucault interpreters who turn the clinical gaze into something deterministic, oppressive and disciplining. Barry argues that the gaze in the clinic is essentially fallible and hence not by definition oppressive.

14. Pappas & Seale 2009.

15. Boonstra et al. (2008) report on an ambitious homecare webcam project in the north of the Netherlands. They report that the implementation of the webcams failed because there was no clear goal described for the end-users: the nurses and the patients at home. In many cases, professionals and patients did not even use the webcam once. The assumed users simply did not know what to use it for.

16. For a subtle analysis of the meanings attached to the home and the way care and technology may interfere with this, see Milligan, Mort & Roberts 2010; Milligan 2009.

17. It would be interesting to know if relational distance could also be 'too close' for the webcam to be of any help. To find this out, research could be done among long-distance lovers using a webcam to keep in (and yet rather 'out of') touch.

18. This may be a variety of the 'pen friend' or 'pen pal', someone with whom to exchange letters without ever meeting them.

Notes Chapter 7

1. How decision makers always relate economic reasoning to some kind of good merits a study in itself. Relating efficiency to goodness might be a heritage of Adam Smith's philosophy of the invisible hand, the mechanism

that turns individual strivings for one's own benefit into a higher, common good. However, this notion is to be preferred to the recent climate of ruthless budget cuts that do not take into account the kind of care that decision-makers are after. From an ethical perspective, it is not enough to account for the abolishment of certain care practices with cost arguments only, unless one is ready to accept a cynical politics in health care. Decision makers should always account for the nature and acceptability of the care practices they are trying to create, by budget cuts or in other ways.

2. For instance, Boonstra et al. (2008) do not do this. They present a tentative cost efficiency analysis with many caveats, calculating efficiency by relating the nurses' rating of the frequency that telecare contacts could be substituted for actual home visits.

3. This is what Zuiderent-Jerak and Van der Grinten (2009) seem to think, even if they suggest a multiplication of markets. However, they construct a market with only two players: the government and producers. Astonishingly, they do not bring professionals into the calculation. Likewise, an analysis of the position of patients would not have hurt the validity of their analysis. Apparently, in their attempt to make the idea of markets more complex, the authors have dramatically reduced the notion of what politics consists of.

4. The reason for this varies depending on whom one is speaking to. Doctors argue that many ICT interventions are not evidence-based and that studies need to show whether quality improvements for patients take place. They accuse busy producers of 'cowboyism' because of the impact of telecare on working processes without a proper outlook on desirable effects. Producers and health care professionals pioneering in telecare accuse doctors of arrogance and conservatism, serving their own happiness rather than their patients. These discussions can become quite ugly. I once witnessed a sort of celebratory 'doctor bashing' at a conference – hardly a hopeful customer-supplier relationship. The government does not want to take the lead and tries to stimulate professionals and producers to do so themselves. The patient has, so far, no 'voice' in this market (Pols 2010b; Pols, Schermer & Willems 2008).

5. The national patient and consumer organisation is organised by the government in the Netherlands. See Trappenburg 2008; Bovenkamp & Trappenburg 2010.

6. Note that this idea of efficiency is to make access to care easier, not to reduce the nurses' workload. The municipality and the homecare organisations finance these projects, without using health care budgets or health insurance.

7. See Boonstra et al. 2008; López & Domènech 2009.

8. Analyses in the literature demonstrating the difficulty of rearranging work practices include May & Ellis 2001; Nicolini 2006; Lehoux et al. 2002.

9. The way a comparable project solved the problem of 'going into the neighbourhood' versus webcamming is by doing all the hands-on care in the morning when people need quick help to start their day, and taking time in the afternoon to do the social chats over the webcam.

10. Note that there is extra work for patients, too. They need to fill in questionnaires that aim to show if there is a change in their quality of life. The patients often see this as part of their treatment.

11. http://www.onderzoekinformatie.nl/nl/oi/nod/onderzoek/OND1298070/.

12. See Pols & Willems 2011 for an extensive discussion of this case.

13. This downplays the importance of 'ethical design' that is promoted in the Netherlands. If devices change when they are put into practice, this should be an area of concern for the ethics of technology as well. For an ethics of design, see Verbeek 2006.

Notes Chapter 8

1. See Marres (2005) for ways in which particular events create particular 'publics'. Professionals and people with chronic disease are an important public for telecare, but they do not have a strong influence on the market.
2. In a personal communication, Amade M'Charek suggested that all care practices should be conceived of as innovative, as they are constantly changing and made to change. I agree with her because, fundamentally, a practice that treats new 'cases' on a daily basis should always improvise. In theory, however, there are rather sleepy care practices as well, where care is given more routinely than elsewhere and outcomes are less 'under construction'. Hence I stick to the term 'innovative care practices' for analytical reasons.
3. For analyses of interactions and unexpected pathways, see Mol 2002; Pols 2003; 2006; M'Charek 2010.
4. This idea of attaining objectivity by excluding human beliefs also existed in the first experimental practices. Boyle undertook his air pump experiments so that 'nature could speak for itself' by producing 'machine-made facts' uncontaminated by any human interest in the outcome of the experiment. Shapin & Schaffer 1985.
5. See Timmermans & Berg 2003.
6. Critical voices argue that this does not work. Results written up by interested industries present the same research more favourably than independent researchers. In the Netherlands this led to critical discussions on the responsibility of the government to control the pharmaceutical industry. See the discussion set in motion after an article in a leading Dutch newspaper, *NRC Handelsblad*, on 21 February 2009 by Trudy Dehue, Professor of Theory and History of Psychology, University of Groningen: '*Onderzoekers die afhankelijk zijn van de farmaceutische industrie ruïneren onze gezondheid* (Researchers dependent on the pharmaceutical industry are ruining our health)'.
7. This puts the doctors in the place of the exotic patients discussed in Chapter 5. They are seen as people with experiential knowledge that is unreliable and often wrong.
8. See Chapter 5, where successful patient participation in medical research was attributed to the context of orphan diseases (Callon & Rabéharisoa 2003), diseases that had not yet gained medical scientists' attention.
9. See Van de Bovenkamp & Trappenburg 2009.
10. See also Struhkamp et al. 2009; Mol 1998; 2010; Moser 2010.
11. Mol 2006, 2008 and Moser 2010 usefully describe this for professionals as a difference between improving and proving.
12. The use of the term 'state-of-the-art' is intentional. There are creative quantitative designs and descriptive statistics that provide useful knowledge for care practices, even if it would wrinkle the 'pure' scientists' noses. It is not

quantification per se that is hard to fit but rather the strict designs' useful quantification demands.

13. See also Langstrup-Nielsen 2005; Finch et al. 2003.

14. For an analysis of how the clinical trial is an intervention, see Dehue 2002; 2004; 2005. Rather than 'mirror nature' to present the 'facts', it is an intervention in a practice. For a critique on the metaphor of mirroring, see Rorty 1979. An innovative technology – e.g. telecare – is not a finite 'intervention' that has predetermined effects that may be assessed in standard research. See May et al. 2001; Lehoux et al. 2002; Nicolini, 2006.

15. Francis Bacon argued that nature should be 'tortured' to give away her secrets. Not being subjective does not mean not shaping one's object. See e.g. Pesic 1999 for an argument against the notion of torture and an idea of *mutual wrestling* between nature and the scientist, which is still a metaphor of violence. Even so, the practice of moulding care practices is problematic when it *damages* care practices.

16. Moser (2010) shows how methods such as video registration of care and ethnography might make visible things that are impossible to articulate by means of clinical trials. May (2006) also shows that the content of the knowledge produced with the help of RCTs is not always helpful for decisions about telecare systems. Together with Finch et al. (2003); they recommend ethnographic studies as suitable for evaluating tele-health care. See also May et al. 2003; Callén et al. 2009. For an impressive demonstration of the use of auto-ethnography that articulates yet different matters of concern in care, see Taylor 2010.

17. That research practices interfere with studied practices is nothing new, and researchers are well aware of this. There is literature on placebo and Hawthorn effects (effects brought about by doing research). In quantum physics it is common knowledge that one's observations influence the object observed; physicists live with this because the deviations are small enough to be able to ignore them. When comparing measurements in Euclidean space with those that include time, as in relativity theory, physicists deem the errors too small to complicate calculations. See Barad 2007. The consequences do not seem to be keeping medical practice researchers awake; it has not changed research practices yet. This may be because the self-understanding of research practices does not highlight these matters. They are anomalies or negligible measuring errors that they do not have to take into account.

18. See Pols 2008. My suggestion is not to contrast subjectivity and objectivity but rather norms and facts. As the book demonstrates, there is a harmonious relation between facts and values. Scientists can make endless varieties in their articulations of any situation. They can talk about a situation on a molecular level, a socio-political level, analyse it in terms of gender relations, pinpoint the historical events that lead up to it, and so on. These articulations are all true, yet all different. *What* articulation works *where* is the normative question.

19. See Kuhn's notion of 'normal science', where methods and questions are taken for granted (Kuhn 1962).

20. There is always some disturbance when doing research. However, ethnographic methods do not directly interfere with the telecare practice as a process. The research takes only the nurse's time; they do not need to collect

data, just tell about their experiences with the project and/or allow the researcher to look on while they are working. These unobtrusive methods do not rigorously shape the object of research but try to trace them in their 'natural habitat'.

21. This is a reference to the idea of 'ontological politics' and Law's ideas on performativity (Mol 1991; Law 2004) or the statement that 'science is politics pursued by other means' (see e.g. Harbers 2005; Latour 1983). In the version suggested here, not only scientists or texts create worlds and subjectivities, care practices also do so. See Moser (2011) for moving theory to new practices.

22. Machiavelli's political philosophy would be a fitting model here. See the analysis by Pitkin 1994.

23. This is a complaint from people who try to 'implement': things do not go nearly as fast as they like and they meet a lot of what they call 'resistance' from the field. My articulation is that the new gadget bumps into existing norms and routines, and people need time to tinker with them or have good reasons to stick to their old ways of doing things. See also Pols 2004, Chapter 7.

24. Note that the work is to describe practices and articulate knowledge from them. This is different from asking opinions of participants, which researchers who measure patient satisfaction often do. Asking for opinions fits the consumer patient I described in Chapter 5. It is obviously easier to measure what people *want* than to articulate what they *know* or what *values* are embedded in their routines. See Pols 2005 for the way in which a politics of positions instead of perspectives may draw in 'patients who do not speak' in research into care. For the work needed to create a perspective, see Velpry 2008.

25. In their wonderful reflections on telecare policy, Callén et al. (2009) analyse the possibilities for users to influence telecare developments through health technology assessment (HTA). First, it is unclear who may represent whom in deliberations about good telecare design. Second, HTA is concerned with design rather than domestication processes and is limited in scope. Third, the differences between expert and lay person are not resolved. As a solution to these dilemmas, Callén and her colleagues propose participatory action research (PAR). PAR implies that users are involved in designing the research, including formulation of research questions, selection of the methodologies and interpretation of the results. This is a great suggestion, although it would not solve the matter of representation completely. I am concerned about the new expertise this demands from users: it demands the expertise of a researcher who is expert at juggling different methodologies and translating them into different questions. The task for users is not only to keep their practice going and 'do the innovative care' besides reflecting on the values and forms of care that are generated. They have to learn how to do multi-method research. In my alternative – uncontrolled field studies – participants may delegate the task of doing research to involved ethnographers. The explicit discussion of the specific *position* created for the users of these practices should guarantee that they are not 'forgotten'. Callén et al. argue for 'giving ears' instead of 'giving voice'; my alternative would be 'making voice' by articulating embodied knowledge. See Finch, Mort, May &

Mair (2005) for an analysis of the (absence of the) influence of patients on the introduction of health care technology.

26. Of course, researchers are not 'independent' in and of themselves. Rather, their dependencies lie elsewhere, for instance in the way research is funded and results get published. In the example, their independence is from the organisations participating in the experiment, including the industry.

27. See e.g. Milligan, Mort & Roberts 2010.

28. This practice is more common in mental health care, at least in the Netherlands, England and the US. See Dixon et al. 1997; Mead et al. 2001; Mowbray et al. 1998; Boevink 2006a. Patients in mental health care have organised themselves as professionals using experiential knowledge. They organise education and training for these professionals-to-be. Any self-respecting long-term mental health care facility employs a couple of these new professionals.

29. To study the effectiveness of a telecare device departs from a deterministic idea of what technology is, making the part of users and contexts invisible because of their assumed irrelevance.

References

Aanestad, M. (2003) The camera as an actor: Design-in-Use of telemedicine infrastructure in surgery. *Computer supported cooperative work*, 12, 1-20.

Akrich, M. (2010) From Communities of Practice to Epistemic Communities: Health Mobilizations on the Internet. *Sociological Research Online*, 15, 2, 10 http://www.socresonline.org.uk/15/2/10.html

Akrich, M. (1992) The De-Scription of technical objects. In: W.E. Bijker & J. Law, *Shaping technology/ building society. Studies in sociotechnical change*. Cambridge (MS), London (GB): The MIT Press, 205-224.

Anderson, W. (2008) *The Collectors of Lost Souls: Turning Kuru Scientists into Whitemen*. Baltimore: Johns Hopkins University Press.

Argyle, M. (1990) *Bodily communication*. London: Routledge.

Arksey, H. (1994) Expert and Lay Participation in the Construction of Medical Knowledge, *Sociology of Health and Illness*, 16, 4, 448-468.

Barad, K. (2007) *Meeting the Universe Halfway: Quantum Physics and the Entanglement of Matter and Meaning*, Durham: Duke University Press.

Barbot J. (2006) How to build an 'active' patient'. *Social Science & Medicine*, 3, 538-51.

Barbot, J. & N. Dodier (2002). Multiplicity in scientific medicine: the experience of HIV-positive patients, *Science, Technology & Human Values*, 27, 404-40.

Barry, A. (1995) Reporting and visualising. In: Jenks, C. (ed.) Visual culture. London: Routledge, 42-57.

Bauer, K. (2004) Cyber medicine and the moral integrity of the physician-patient relationship. *Ethics and information technology*, 6, 83-91.

Benatar, S.R. (2001) Distributive Justice and Clinical Trials in the Third World. *Theoretical Medicine* 22, 169-76.

Berg, M. (2002) Patients and professionals in the information society: what might keep us awake in 2013. *International Journal of Medical Informatics*, 66, 31-7.

Berg, M. (1997). Rationalizing Medical Work. Cambridge, Mass: MIT Press.

Berker, T., Hartmann, M., Punie, Y. & Ward, K.J. (2006) Domestication of media and technology. Maidenhead: Open University Press.

Blumer, H. (1954). What is wrong with social theory? *American Sociological Review*, 18, 3-10.

Boevink, W. (2006b) From being a disorder to dealing with life. *Schizophrenia Bulletin*, 1, 2.

Boevink, W. (ed.) (2006a). *Stories of recovery. Working together towards experiential knowledge in mental health care*. Utrecht: Trimbos-instituut.

Boltanski L. & Thévenot L. (1991) *De la justifications. Les économies de la grandeur.* Editions Gallimard.

Boonstra, A., Broekhuis, M., Offenbeek, M. van, Westerman, W. Wijngaard, J. Wortman, H. (2008) *Kijken op afstand. Op zoek naar de effectiviteit en efficiency van Koala telecare en telecare*. Publieksversie van het eindrapport RuG/RHO: 'Kijken op afstand, een leerzaam alternatief' Groningen: RuG/RHO. http://www.zorginnovatieforum.nl/projecten/ZoA/Koala eindrapport.pdf, last consulted 29 oktober 2009.

Borup, M. Brown, N., Konrad, K. & Van Lente, H. (2006) The sociology of expectations in science and technology. *Technology analysis & strategic management*, 18, 285-98.

Bovenkamp, H.M. Van de, & Trappenburg, M.J. (2010) Government Influence on Patient Organizations, *Health Care Analysis*, DOI 10.1007/s10728-010-0155-7

Bovenkamp, H.M. Van de, Trappenburg, M.J. & Grit, K.J. (2010) Patient participation in collective health care decision making: The Dutch model. *Health Expectations*, 13, 73-85.

Bovenkamp, H.M. van de & Trappenburg, M.J. (2009) Reconsidering patient participation in guideline development. *Health Care Analysis*, 17, 198-216.

Bowen, G.A. (2006) Grounded Theory and Sensitizing Concept. *International Journal of Qualitative Methods*, 5 (3), www.ualberta.ca/~iiqm/backissues/5_3/pdf/bowen.pdf

Bowker, G.C. (2006) Memory practices in the sciences (inside technology). Cambridge, MA: MIT Press.

Brandt, A.M. (1978) Racism and Research: The Case of the Tuskegee Syphilis Study – The Hastings Center Report, Vol. 8, No. 6 (Dec., 1978), pp. 21-29

Brown, H. (2010) 'If we sympathise with them, they'll relax' Fear/respect and medical care in a Kenyan hospital. *Medische Antropologie*. Special issue: 'Care and Health Care', in: Hiddinga, A., Pols, J., Trakas, D. & Van der Geest, S. (theme editors) 22,1, 125-42.

Brown, N. & Michael, M. (2003) A sociology of expectations. Retrospecting prospects and prospecting retrospects. *Technology Analysis & Strategic Management*, 15, 3-18.

Brown, N. (2003). Hope against hype - accountability in biopasts, presents and futures. *Science Studies*, 16(2), 3-21

Callén, B., Domenèch, M., López, D. & Tirado, F. (2009) Telecare research: (cosmo)politicizing methodology. *Alter. European Journal of Disability Research*, 3, 110-22.

Callon, M. & Rabeharisoa, V. (2008) The growing engagement of emergent concerned groups in political and economic life. Lessons from the French Association of Neuromuscular Disease Patients. *Science, Technology & Human Values*, 33, 230-61.

Callon, M. & Rabeharisoa, V. (2004) Articulating bodies: The case of muscular dystrophies, (unpublished paper).

Callon, M., Rabeharisoa, V. (2003), Research 'in the wild' and the shaping of new social identities, *Technology in Society, Studies in Science, Technology, and Society (STS) North and South*, 2, 193-204.

Callon, M. & Rabeharisoa V. (2002) The involvement of patients' associations in research. Unesco, Blackwell publishers, 57-65.

Callon, M. (2005) Disabled persons of all countries, unite! In: Latour, B. & Wiebel, P. *Making things public. Atmospheres of Democracy*, Karlsruhe: ZKM, Center for Art and Media, Cambridge (Mass) and London: The MIT Press, 308-13.

Callon, M. (1999) The role of lay people in the production and dissemination of scientific knowledge. *Science, Technology & Society*, 4, 81-94.

Callon, M. (1985) Some elements of a sociology of translation: domestication of the scallops and the fishermen of St. Brieu Bay, In Law, J. (ed.) *Power, Action and Belief. Sociological Review Monograph.* London: Routledge and Kegan Paul, 196-223.

Callon, M. and Law, J. (1982) On interests and their transformation: enrollment and counter enrollment, *Social Studies of Science*, 12, 615-25.

Canguilhem, G. (1966) *The normal and the pathological.* New York: Zone Books 1989.

Cartwright, L. (2000). Reach out and heal someone: telemedicine and the globalization of health care. *Health*, 4, 3, 347-77.

Charmaz, K. (2003). Grounded theory: Objectivist and constructivist methods. In N.K. Denzin & Y.S. Lincoln (Eds.), *Strategies for qualitative inquiry.* Thousand Oaks, CA: Sage, 249-291.

Charmaz, K. (2000). Experiencing chronic illness. Fitzpatrick R. & Scrimshaw, SC, *Handbook of social studies in health and medicine*, London: Sage, 277-92.

Clutton-Brock, J. (ed) (1988) *The Walking Larder: Patterns of Domestication, Pastoralism, and Predation*, London: Unwin Hyam.

Cohen, M.Z., Tripp-Reimer, T., Smith, C., Sorofman, B., and Lively, S. (1994) Explanatory Models of Diabetes: Patient Practitioner Variation. *Social Science and Medicine*, 38, 1, 59-66.

Cooley, D.R. (2001) Distributive Justice and Clinical Trials in the Third World. *Theoretical Medicine*, 22, 151-67.

Corbin, J. & A. Strauss (1988) *Unending work and care: Managing chronic illness at home.* San Francisco: Jossey Bass University Press.

Cukor, P. and Baer, L. (1994) Human factors issues in telemedicine: a practical guide with particular attention to psychiatry. *Telemedicine Today*, 29, 16-18.

Currell R., C. Urquhart, P. Wainwright P. et al. (2000) *Telemedicine versus face tot face patient care: effects on professional practice and health care outcomes.* Chichester: John Wiley & Sons, The Cochrane Library.

Dehue, T. (2008) *De depressie-epidemie. De geschiedenis van neerslachtigheid.* Amsterdam: Augustus.

Dehue, T. (2005). History of the Control Group. In: Everitt, B. and Howell, D. (eds) *Encyclopedia of Statistics in the Behavioral Science*, Chichester, UK: Wiley, 2, 829-836

Dehue, T. (2004). Historiography taking issue. Analyzing an experiment with heroin maintenance. *Journal of the History of the Behavioral Sciences*, 40, 3, 247-265.

Dehue, T. (2002). A Dutch treat. Randomized controlled experimentation and the case of heroin-maintenance in the Netherlands. *History of the Human Sciences*, 15, 2, 75-98.

Department of Health (2001) *The Expert Patient: A New Approach to Chronic Disease Management for the 21st Century*, Department of Health, London.

Dixon L., A. Hackman & A. Lehman (1997) Consumers as Staff in Assertive Community Treatment Program, *Administration and Policy in Mental Health*, 25, 199-208.

Donner, J. The Rules of Beeping: Exchanging Messages Using Missed Calls on Mobile Phones in sub-Saharan Africa. Paper presented at the annual meeting of the International Communication Association, Sheraton New York, New York City, NY, 2009-05-25

Dunn, E., Conrath, D., Acton, H., Higgins, C. Matha, M. & Bain, H. (1980) Tele-medicine links patients in Sioux Lookout with doctors in Toronto. *Canadian Medical Association Journal*, 122, 23, 484-487.

Edgar, A. (2005) The expert patient. Illness as practice. *Medicine, Health Care & Philosophy*, 8, 165-71.

Eisenberg L. (1977) Disease and illness. Distinctions between professional and popular ideas of sickness. *Culture, Medicine & Psychiatry*, 1, 1, 9-23

Eminovic, N., De Keizer, N.F., Bindels, P.J.E. & Hasman, A. (2007) Maturity of teledermatology evaluation research: a systematic literature review. *British Journal of Dermatology*, 156, 412-9.

Epstein, S. (1996) *Impure Science. Aids, activism and the politics of knowledge*, Berkeley: University of California Press.

Epstein, S. (2008) Patient groups and Health movements. in: Hacket, E.J., Amsterdamska, O., Lynch, M., Wajcman, J. (eds) *The Handbook of science and technology studies*. Cambridge: MIT press.499-539.

Epstein, S. (1995) The construction of lay expertise: AIDS activism and the forging of credibility in the reform of clinical trials, *Science, Technology & Human Values*, 20, 4, 408-37.

Estrada, M., Balasch, M. & Vayreda, A. (in preparation), 'Follow the treatment and get as much information as you can': A qualitative study of information management in a virtual patient community.

Evans-Pritchard, E.E. 1937. *Witchcraft, Oracles and Magic Among the Azande*. Clarendon Press.

Finch, T., Mort, M., May, C. & Mair, F. (2005) Telecare; perspectives on the changing role of patients and citizens. *Journal of Telemedicine and Telecare*, 11, Supplement 1, S1:51-3.

Finch, T., May, C., Mair, F., Mort, M. & Gask, L. (2003) Integrating service development with evaluation in telehealthcare: an ethnographic study. *British Medical Journal*, 327, 1205-9.

Fischer, C.S. (1992) *America Calling: A Social History of the Telephone to 1940*. Berkeley, LA: University of California Press.

Fisk, M.J. (1997) Telecare equipment in the home. Issues of intrusiveness and control. *Journal of Telemedicine and Telecare*, 3, Supplement 1, 30-2.

Fisk, M.J. (1998) Telecare at home: factors influencing technology choices and user acceptance. *Journal of Telemedicine and Telecare*, 4, 80-3.

Foucault, M. (1973) *The Birth of the Clinic: An Archaeology of Medical Perception*. London: Tavistock publications.

Foucault, M. (1971). *L'ordre du Discourse*. Paris: Gallimard.

Foucault, M. (1977) *Discipline and Punish: The Birth of the Prison*. New York: Random House.

Gad, C. & Bruun-Jensen, C. (2010) On the Consequences of Post-ANT. *Science, Technology, & Human Values*, 36, 5, 55-80

Gammon, D, Sörlie, T., Bergvik, S., & Sörensen Höifödt, T. (1998) Psychotherapy supervision conducted via videoconferencing: a qualitative study of users' experiences. *Nordic Journal of Psychiatry*, 52, 411-21.

Gourlay, S. (2002) Tacit knowledge, tacit knowing or behaving? Paper presented at the 3rd European Organizational Knowledge, Learning, and Capabilities Conference, Athens, 5-6 April.

Gourlay, S. (2006) Towards conceptual clarity for 'tacit knowledge': a review of empirical studies, *Knowledge Management Research & Practice*, 4, 60-69

Greatbatch, D. Hanlon, G. Goode, J. O'Cathain, A. Strangleman, D. Luff, D. (2005) Telephone triage, expert systems and clinical expertise. *Sociology of Health & Illness*, 27, 6, 802-830

Greenhalgh, T. (2009) Patient and public involvement in chronic illness: beyond the expert patient. *BMJ*, 338, 629-31.

Haas, P.M. (1992) 'Banning Chlorofluorocarbons: Epistemic Community Efforts to Protect Stratospheric Ozone', *International Organization*, 46, 1, 187-244.

Habermas, J. (1985) *Theorie des Kommunikativen Handelns. Handlungsrationalität und gesellschaftliche Rationalisierung*. Frankfurt am Main: Suhrkamp Verlag.

Habraken, J.M., Pols, J., Bindels, P.J.E. & Willems, D.L. (2008) The silence of patients with end-stage COPD: an qualitative study. *British Journal of General Practice*, 58, 844-9.

Haraway, D. (1991) *Simians, cyborgs, and women. The reinvention of nature*. London: Free Association Books.

Haraway, D. (1991). Situated Knowledges: The science question in feminism and the privilege of partial perspective. In: *Simians, cyborgs and women. The reinvention of nature*. New York: Routledge.

Haraway, D. (2008) *When species meet*. University of Minnesota Press.

Harbers, H. (2005) Epilogue: Political Materials – Material politics. In: Harbers, H. (ed.) *Inside the politics of technology. Agency and normativity in the co-production of technology and society*. Amsterdam: Amsterdam University Press, 257-272.

Hart, A. Henwood, F. & Wyatt, S. (2004) The Role of the Internet in Patient-Practitioner Relationships: Findings from a Qualitative Research Study. *Journal of Medical Internet Research*, 6, 3, e36.

Healy, D. (2002) The Creation of Psychopharmacology. Cambridge, Mass: Harvard University Press.

Hendriks, R (1998) Egg timers, human values and the care of autistic youths. *Science, Technology & Human Values*, 23, 4, 399-424.

Henry, S.G. (2010) Polanyï's tacit knowing and the relevance of epistemology to clinical medicine. *Journal of Evaluation in Clinical Practice*, 16, 292-7.

Henwood, F., Wyatt, S., Hart, A. & Smith, J. (2003) 'Ignorance is bliss sometimes': constraints on the emergence of the 'informed patient' in the changing landscapes of health information. *Sociology of Health & Illness*, 25, 6, 589-607.

Hester, J.S. (2005) Bricolage and bodies of knowledge: exploring consumer responses to controversies about the third generation oral contraceptive pill. *Body & Society*, 11, 77-95

Hughes, B. & Paterson, K. The social model of disability and the disappearing body. Towards a sociology op impairment. *Disability & Society*, 12, 3, 325-40.

Hughes, B. (2009) Wounded/ monstrous /abject: a critique of the disabled body in the sociological imaginary. *Disability & Society*, 24, 4, 399-410.

Hunter, K.M. (1991) *Doctors' stories: the narrative structure of medical knowledge*. Princeton: Princeton University Press.

Hutchins, E. (1995) *Cognition in the wild*. Cambridge, MA: MIT press.

Ihde, D. (1990) Technology and the Lifeworld. Bloomington/ Minneapolis: Indiana University Press.

Johnson, K. (2006) TV Screen, Not Couch, Is Required for This Session, *New York Times*, 8 June 2006.

Jonssen, A.R. & S. Toulmin, (1988) *The Abuse of Casuistry: A History of Moral Reasoning*. Chicago: University of Chicago Press.

Kammen, J. van (ed.) (2002) *Zorgtechnologie, kansen voor innovatie en gebruik*. (Care technology, chances for innnovation and use) Den Haag: Stichting Toekomstbeeld der Techniek (STT).

Kivits, J. (2004) Researching the 'informed patient'. The case of online health information seekers. *Information, Communication & Society*, 7, 4, 510-30.

Kleinman, A. (1980) *Patients and Healers in the Context of Culture*. Berkeley: University of California Press.

Kleinman, A. & Van der Geest, S. (2009) Care in healthcare: Remaking the moral world of medicine. *Medische Antropologie*, 21: 159-68.

Knudsen, C. (2002).Video mediated communication: Producing a sense of presence between individuals in shared virtual reality. In: J. Baggaley, P. Fahy & C. O'Hagan (Eds.), *Educational Conferencing: Video and text traditions*. Proceedings of the First International Symposium on Educational Conferencing (ISEC), Banff, Alberta, co-sponsored by Athabasca University and the Social Sciences and Humanities Research Council of Canada. Retrieved May 12, 2004, from http://cde.athabascau.ca/ISEC2002/

Korsten, J.P.A.M. (2010) Impact of Remote Support on Patients receiving Palliative Care. 'Investigation into the impact of the Health Buddy on patients receiving palliative chemotherapy who have a prognosis of at least six months' Masters thesis for Health Services Innovation, Faculty of Health, Medicine and Life Sciences, Maastricht University.

Kuhn, T.S. (1962) *The Structure of Scientific Revolutions*, Chicago: Univ. of Chicago Press.

Langstrup, H. (2008) Making connections through online asthma monitoring. *Chronic Illness*, 4, 118-126.

Langstrup-Nielsen, H.L. (2005): Linking Healthcare – An inquiry into the changing performances of web-based technology for asthma monitoring. PhD thesis, Copenhagen Business School.

Latour, B. (1992) Where are the missing masses? The sociology of a few mundane artifacts. In: W.E. Bijker & J. Law, *Shaping technology/ building society. Studies in sociotechnical change*. Cambridge (MS), London (GB): The MIT Press, 225-258.

Latour, B. (1999) *Pandora's Hope: Essays on the Reality of Science Studies*, Cambridge, Mass., Harvard University Press.

Latour, B. (1996) *Aramis or the love of technology*. Cambridge: Harvard University Press, 1996.

Latour, B. (1991) On recalling ANT. In: In: Law, J., Hassard J. (eds). Actor Network Theory and After. Oxford: Blackwell Publishers, 15-24.

Latour, B. (1987) *The Pasteurization of French Society*. Cambridge MA: MIT Press.

Latour, B. (1983) Give me a laboratory and I will raise the world. in: Knorr-Cetina, K. & Mulkay, M. (eds) *Science observed. Perspectives on the social studies of Science.* London: Sage, 141-70.

Law, J. (1994) *Organising Modernity.* Oxford: Blackwell Publishers.

Law, J. (1999). After ANT: complexity, naming and topology. In: Law, J., Hassard J. (eds). *Actor Network Theory and After.* Oxford: Blackwell Publishers, 1-14.

Law, J. (2004) *After Method: Mess in Social Science Research.* Durham & London: Duke University Press.

Law, J. and Mol, A. (2008). The Actor-Enacted: Cumbrian Sheep in 2001. in: Knappet, C. & Malafouris L. (eds) *Material Agency: Towards a Non-Anthropocentric Approach.* New York, Springer, 57-77.

Law, J. (1997) Traduction/ trahison: notes on ANT. Published by the Department of Sociology, Lancaster University at: http://lancaster.ac.uk/sociology/stslaw2.html.

Law, J. (1987) Technology, closure and heterogeous engineering: the case of the Portugese expansion. In Bijker, W. Pinch, T. and Hughes, T.P. (eds) *The Social Construction of Technological Systems,* Cambridge MA: MIT Press.

Lederer, S. E. (1995) Subjected to Science: Human Experimentation in America before the Second World War. Baltimore, MD: Johns Hopkins University Press.

Lehman, P. (ed.) (2004) *Coming off Psychiatric Drugs. Successful Withdrawal from Neuroleptics, Antidepressants, Lithium, Carbamazepine and Tranquilizers.* Shrewsbury: Peter Lehman Publishing.

Lehoux, P. Sicotte, C. Denis, J.L., Berg, M. & Lacroix, A. (2002) The theory of use behind telemedicine: how compatible with physicians' clinical routines? *Social Science & Medicine,* 54, 889-904.

Lettinga, A., & Mol, A. (1999). Clinical specificity and the non-generalities of science: On innovation strategies for neurological physical therapy. *Theoretical Medicine and Bioethics,* 10, 6, 517-535.

Lettinga, A. (2000) Diversity in neurological physiotherapy. A comparative analysis of clinical and scientific practices. Groningen: Northern Centre for Healthcare Research.

Lévi-Strauss, C. (1966) *The Savage mind.* Chicago: University of Chicago Press.

Lichtenstein, G. (2010) Vicuña conservation and poverty alleviation? Andean communities and international fibre markets, *International journal of the commons.* 4, 1, available at: . Date accessed: 11 Oct. 2011.

Lie, M. & Sörensen, K.H. (1996) *Making Technology our own? Domesticating technology into everyday life.* Oslo: Scandinavian University Press.

López, D. & Domènech, M. (2008) On inscriptions and ex-inscriptions: the production of immediacy in a home telecare service. *Environment and Planning D: Society and Space,* 26, 663-75.

López, D. & Domènech, M. (2009) Embodying autonomy in a Home Telecare Service. *The Sociological Review,* 56, 181-95.

López, D., Callén, B., Tirado, F. y Domènech, M. (2010) How to become a guardian angel. Providing Safety in a Home Telecare Service. In: Mol, A., Moser, I. & Pols, J. (eds.) *Care in Practice. On Tinkering in clinics, homes and farms.* Bielefeld: Transcript Verlag, 73-92.

López, D. (2010) The Securitzation of Care Spaces: Lessons from telecare. In: M. Schillmeier and Domènech (eds), *New Technologies and Emerging Spaces of Care.* Farnham: Ashgate, 40-55.

Lupton, D. (1997) Consumerism, reflexivity and the medical encounter, *Social Science & Medicine*, 24, 3, 373-81.

Marres, N. (2005) No Issue, No Public: Democratic Deficits after the Displacement of Politics, PhD dissertation, University of Amsterdam, 2005, http://dare.uva.nl/document/17061

May, C., Rapley, T., Moreira, T., Finch, T. & Heaven, B. (2006) Technogovernance: evidence, subjectivity and the clinical encounter in primary care medicine. *Social Science & Medicine*, 62, 1022-30.

May, C., Finch, T., Mair, F., Ballini, L., Dowrick, C., Eccles, M., Gask, L., MacFarlane, A., Murray, E. Rapley, T., Rogers, A., Treweek, S., Wallace, P., Anderson, G., Burns, J., & Heaven, B. (2007). Understanding the implementation of complex interventions in health care: the normalization process model. *BMC Health Services Research*. 19, 7, 148.

May, C. (2006) Mobilising modern facts: health technology assessment and the politics of evidence. *Sociology of Health & Illness*, 28, 5, 513-532.

May, C. Finch, T. Mair, F. & Mort, M. (2005) Towards a wireless patient. Chronic illness, scarce care and technological innovation in the United Kingdom. *Social Science & Medicine*, 61, 7, 1485-94.

May, C., Mort, M., Williams, T., Mair, F. & Gask, L. (2003) Health technology assessment in its local contexts: studies of telehealthcare. *Social Science & Medicine*, 57, 4, 697-710.

May, C., Gask, L., Atkinson, T., Ellis, N., Mair, F. & Esmail, A. (2001) Resisting and promoting new technologies in clinical practice: the case of telepsychiatry. *Social Science & Medicine*, 52, 12, 1889-1901.

May, C. & Ellis, N.T. (2001) When protocols fail: technical evaluation, biomedical knowledge and the social productions of 'facts' about a telemedicine clinic. *Social Science and Medicine*, 53, 989-1002.

M'charek, A. (2010a) Fragile Differences, Relational Effects: Stories about the Materiality of Race and Sex, *European Journal of Women's Studies*, 17, 4, 1-16.

M'charek, A. (2010b) When whiteness becomes a problem. (Un)doing differences in the case of Down's Syndrome. *Medische Antropologie*, 22, 263-76.

Mead, S., Hilton, D. & Curtis, L. (2001) Peer support: a theoretical perspective. *Psychiatric Rehabilitation Journal*, 25,2, 134-41.

Miller, J.F. (2006) Opportunities and obstacles for good work in nursing. *Nursing Ethics*, 13, 5, 471-87.

Milligan, C. (2009) *There's No Place like Home: People, Place and Care in an ageing society*. Aldershot: Ashgate Geographies Health Book Series.

Milligan, C., Roberts, C., Mort, M. & Moser, I. (2006) MEDUSE Policy Paper: the Emergence of New Technologies and Responsibilities for Health Care at Home in Europe, www.csi.ensmp.fr/WebCSI/MEDUSE/.

Milligan, C., Roberts, C. & Mort, M. (2010) Telecare and older people: Who cares where? *Social Science & Medicine*, doi: 10.1016/j.socscimed.2010.08.014.

Milligan, C, Mort, M. & Roberts, C. (2010) Cracks in the door? Technology and the shifting topology of care. In: Schillmeier, M. and Domènech, M. (Eds.) *New Technologies and Emerging Spaces of Care*. Farnham: Ashgate, 19-37 .

Miscione, G. (2007) Telemedicine in the upper amazon: interplay with local health care practices. *MIS Quarterly*, 31, 2, 403-425.

Mol, A., Moser, I. & Pols, J. (2010) Care: Putting practice into theory. In: Mol, A. Moser, I. & Pols, J. (eds) *Care in practice. On tinkering in clinics, homes and farms.* Bielefeld: Transcript Verlag. 7-26.

Mol, A. (2010) Care and its values. Good food in the nursing home. In: Mol, A., Moser, I. & Pols, J. (eds) *Care in practice. On tinkering in clinics, homes and farms.* Bielefeld: Transcript Verlag, 215-34.

Mol, A. (2008) *The logic of care.* London: Routledge.

Mol, A. & Karayalcin, C. (2008) 'Evidence' is niet genoeg; kanttekeningen uit de praktijk van de acute psychiatrie, *Tijdschrift Voor Psychiatrie,* 50, 359-364.

Mol, A. (2006) Proving or improving: On health care research as a form of self-reflection. *Qualitative Health Research,* 16, 405-414.

Mol A. & Law, J. (2004) Embodied action, enacted bodies. The example hypoglycaemia. *Body & Society,* 10, 43-62.

Mol, A. (2002) *The body multiple. Ontology in medical practice.* Durham and London: Duke University Press.

Mol, A. (2000) Dit is geen programma. Over empirische filosofie. (This is not a program. On empirical Philosophy) *Krisis,* 1, 1, 6-26. www.krisis.eu/content/2000-1/2000-1-03-mol.pdf

Mol, A. and Berg M. (1998). An Introduction. In: Mol A. and Berg M. (eds) *Differences in Medicine: Unravelling Practices, Techniques and Bodies.* Durham, NCa. and London: Duke University Press, 1-12.

Mol, A. (1998) Missing Links, Making Links. The Performance of some Atheroscleroses, in: Berg, M. and Mol, A. (eds) *Differences in Medicine: Unraveling Practices, Techniques and Bodies.* Durham, London: Duke University Press, 144-65.

Mol, A. (1991) Ontological politics. A word and some questions. In: Law, J., Hassard J. (eds) *Actor Network Theory and After.* Oxford: Blackwell Publishers, 74-89.

Moreira, T. (2006) Heterogeneity and Coordination of Blood Pressure in Neurosurgery. *Social Studies of Science,* 36, 1, 69-97.

Moreira, T. (2004) Self, Agency and the Surgical Collective: detachment. *Sociology of Health & Illness,* 26, 1, 32-49.

Mort, M., May, C. & Williams, T. (2003). Remote doctors and absent patients: Acting at a distance in telemedicine? *Science, Technology and Human Values,* 28, 2, pp. 274-295.

Mort, M., Finch, T. & May, C. (2009) Making and unmaking telepatients. Identity and governance in new health technologies. *Science, Technology & Human Values,* 34, 9-33.

Moser, I. (2011) Dementia and the Limits to Life: Anthropological Sensibilities, STS Interferences, and Possibilities for Action in Care, *Science, Technology & Human Values,* DOI: 10.1177/0162243910396349.

Moser, I. (2009) A body that matters? The role of embodiment in the recomposition of life after a road traffic accident. *Scandinavian Journal of Disability Research,* 11, 2, 81-96

Moser, I. (2010) Perhaps tears should not be counted but wiped away. On quality and improvement in dementia care. In: Mol, A.Moser, I. & Pols, J. (eds) *Care in practice. On tinkering in clinics, homes and farms.* Bielefeld: Transcript verlag, 277-300.

Moser, I. (2006) Disability and the promise of technology: Technology, subjectivity and embodiment within an order of the normal. *Information, Communication and Society*, 9, 3, 373-95.

Moser, I. (2005) On becoming disabled and articulating alternatives: the multiple modes of ordering disability and their interferences, *Cultural Studies*, 19, 667-700.

Moser, I. & Law, J. (1999) Good passages, bad passages. In Law, J., Hassard J. (eds) *Actor Network Theory and After*. Oxford: Blackwell Publishers, 196-219.

Mowbray, C.T., D. Mosley & M.E. Collins (1998) Consumers as Mental Health Providers: First Person Accounts of Benefits and Limitations, *Journal of Behavioral Health Services & Research*, 25, 397-411.

Nettleton, S., Burrows, R., O'Malley, L. & Watt, I. (2004) Health E-Types? An analysis of the everyday use of the Iternet for health. *Information, Communication & Society*, 7, 4, 531-53.

Nicolini, D. (2006) The work to make telemedicine work: a social and articulative view. *Social Science & Medicine*, 62, 2754-67

Nijhof, G. (2001) Ziekenwerk. Een kleine sociologie van alledaags ziekenleven. Amsterdam: Aksant.

Norman, S., (2006) The use of telemedicine in psychiatry. *Journal of psychiatric and mental health nursing* , 13, 771-7.

Onor, M.L. & Misan, S. (2005) The clinical interview and the doctor-patient relationship in telemedicine. *Telemedicine and e-health*, 11, 102-5.

Osborne, T. (2002) Medicine and epistemology: Michel Foucault and the liberality of clinical reason. *History of the human sciences*, 5,2, 63-93.

Oudshoorn, N. (2009) Physical and digital proximity: emerging ways of health care in face-to-face and telemonitoring of heart-failure patients. *Sociology of Health & Illness*, 31, 3, 390-405.

Oudshoorn, N., & Pinch, T. (2003) *How Users Matter: The Co-construction of Users and Technology*. Cambridge: MIT Press.

Polanyi, M. (1966) The tacit dimension. Doubleday 1966.

Pappas, Y. & Seale, C. (2009) The opening phase of telemedicine consultations. An analysis of interaction, *Social Science & Medicine*, 68, 1229-37.

Pesic, P. (1999) Wrestling with Proteus: Francis Bacon and the 'Torture' of Nature. Isis, 90, 1, 81-94.

Petryna, A., Lakoff, A. & Kleinman, A. (eds.) (2006) *Global Pharmaceuticals: Ethics, Markets, Practices*. Durham, NC: Duke University Press.

Petryna, A. (2007) 'Clinical Trials Offshored: On Private Sector Science and Public Health.' *BioSocieties*, 2, 21-40.

Petryna, A. (2009) When Experiments Travel: Clinical Trials and the Global Search for Human Subjects. Princeton: Princeton University Press.

Pickering, A. (1992) Science as Practice and Culture. Chicago & London: University of Chicago Press.

Pitkin, H.F. (1984) *Fortune is a Woman. Gender and Politics in the Thought of Nicollò Machiavelli*. Berkeley, Los Angeles, London: University of California Press.

Pols, J. & Willems, D. (2011) Innovation and Evaluation. About taming and unleashing telecare technologies. *Sociology of Health and Illness*, 33, 4, 484-498.

Pols, J. (2010a) Breathtaking practicalities: A politics of embodied patient positions, *Scandinavian Journal of Disability Research*, DOI: 10.1080/15017419.2010.490726

Pols, J. (2010b) What patients care for with telecare. In: Mol, A. Moser, I. & Pols, J. (eds) Care in practice. On tinkering in clinics, homes and farms. Bielefeld: Transcript verlag, 171-94.

Pols, J. (2010c) Wonderful webcams. About active gazes and invisible technologies. *Science Technology & Human Values*, 36, 2, 1-23.

Pols, J. (2010d) Bringing bodies – and health care – back in. Exploring practical knowledge for living with chronic disease. *Medische Antropologie*, 22, 2, 413-27.

Pols, J. & M'charek (2010a) Introduction. Where are the missing bodies? Disability Studies in the Netherlands. *Medische Antropologie*, 22, 2, 217-224.

Pols, J. & M'charek (guest-editors) (2010b) The body in Disability Studies, special issue of: *Medische Antropologie*, 22, 2.

Pols, J. & Moser, I. (2009) Cold technologies versus warm care? On affective and social relations with and through care technologies, ALTER, European Journal of Disability Research 3 (2009) 159-178.

Pols, J. (2009) The heart of the matter. About good nursing and telecare. Health Care Analysis. An *International Journal of Health Care Philosophy and Policy*, 10.1007/s10728-009-0140-1.

Pols, J. (2008) which empirical research, whose ethics? Articulating ideals in long-term mental health care. In: Widdershoven, G., Hope, T., Van der Scheer, L. & McMillan, J. (editors) *Empirical Ethics in Psychiatry*. Oxford University Press, 51-68.

Pols, J., Schermer, M. & Willems, D. (2008) Telezorgvisie Essay over ontwikkelingen en beloften van telezorg in de Nederlandse gezondheidszorg. (Telecare visions. Essay on the developments and promises of telecare in Dutch health care) Amsterdam: Academic Medical Centre.

Pols, J. (2006) Washing the citizen: washing, cleanliness and citizenship in mental health care. *Culture, Medicine & Psychiatry*, 30, 1, 77-104.

Pols, J. (2005) Enacting appreciations: beyond the patient perspective. *Health Care Analysis*, 13, 3, 203-221.

Pols, J. (2004) Chapter 7: Conclusion: Enacting improvement. In: *Good care. Enacting a complex ideal in long-term psychiatry*. Utrecht: Trimbos-reeks, 149-55, http://www.trimbos.nl/webwinkel/productoverzicht-webwinkel/feiten–cij-fers–beleid/af/afo519-good-care

Pols, J. (2003) Enforcing patient rights or improving care? The interference of two modes of doing good in mental health care, *Sociology of Health & Illness*, 25, 3, 320-347.

Prior, L. (2003) Belief, knowledge and expertise. The emergence of the lay expert in medical sociology. *Sociology of Health & Illness*, 25, 41-57.

Proctor, R. (1988) *Racial Hygiene: Medicine under the Nazis*. Cambridge: Harvard University Press.

Raad voor de Volksgezondheid en Zorg (RVZ) (2010) Gezondheid 2.0. (Health 2.0) Den Haag; RVZ.

Reverby, S.M. (2000) *Examining Tuskegee: The Infamous Syphilis Study and Its Legacy*. Chapel Hill, NC: University of North Carolina Press.

Reverby, S.M. (ed.) (2009) *Tuskegee's Truths: Rethinking the Tuskegee Syphilis Study.* Chapel Hill, NC: University of North Carolina Press.

Roberge, F.A., Pagé, G., Sylvestre, J. & Chahlauoui, J. (1982) Telemedicine in northern Quebec, *Canadian Medical Association Journal*, 127, 8, 707-709.

Roberts, C. & Mort, M. (2009) Reshaping what counts as care: Older people, work and new Technologies Alter, *European Journal of Disability research*, 3, 2, 138-58.

Rorty, R. (1979) *Philosophy and the Mirror of Nature.* Princeton, NJ: Princeton University Press.

Ross Winthereik, B. & Langstrup, H. (2010) When patients care (too much) for information. In: Mol, A., Moser, I. & Pols, J. (eds) *Care in practice. On tinkering in clinics, homes and farms.* Bielefeld: Transcript Verlag, 27-56.

Sacks, O. (1984) *A Leg to Stand On.* New York: Touchstone Books.

Sävenstedt, S., Zingmark, K., Hydén, L.C. & Brulin, C. (2005) Establishing joint attention in remote talks with the elderly about health: a study of nurses' conversation with elderly persons in teleconsultations. *Scandinavian Journal of the Caring Sciences*, 19, 317-24.

Sävenstedt, S., Zingmark, K. and Sandman, P.O. (2004) Being present in a distant room: Aspects of teleconsultations with older people in a nursing home. *Qualitative Health Research*, 14, 1046-1057.

Schermer, M. (2009) Telecare and self-management: opportunity to change the paradigm? *Journal of Medical Ethics*, 35, 688-691.

Schillmeier, M. and Domènech, M. (eds.) (2010) *New Technologies and Emerging Spaces of Care.* Farnham: Ashgate.

Sehon, S.R. & Stanley, D.E. (2003) A philosophical analysis of the evidence-based medicine debate *BMC Health Services Research*, 3, 14,www.biomedcentral. com/1472-6963/3/14.

Shakespeare, T. (2006) *Disability rights and wrongs.* London: Routledge.

Shapin, S. & Schaffer, S.(1985) *Leviathan and the air-pump. Hobbes, Boyle and the experimental life.* Princeton: Princetone University Press.

Silverstone, R. (2005) Domesticating Domestication. Reflections on the Life of Concept, in: Berker, M. Hartmann, Y. Punie and K.Ward (eds) *Domestication of Media and Technologies*, 229-48. Maidenhead: Open University Press.

Silverstone, R., Hirsch, E. and Morley, D. (1992) 'Information and Communication Technologies and the Moral Economy of the Household', in R. Silverstone and E. Hirsch (eds) *Consuming Technologies: Media and Information in Domestic Spaces.* London: Routledge, 115-31.

Sluiter, L. (2007) Virtuele hulpverlener in huiskamer [the virtual living room], *Psy*, 4, p.15.

Smith, K.V. & Godfrey, N.S. (2002) Being a good nurse and doing the right thing: a qualitative study. *Nursing Ethics*, 9, 3, 301-12.

Sparrow, R. (2002) The march of the robot dogs. *Ethics & Information Technology*, 4: 305-18.

Sparrow, R. & L. Sparrow (2006) In the hands of machines? The future of aged care. *Mind Match*,16: 141-61.

Struhkamp, R. Mol, A. & Swierstra, T. (2009) Dealing with In/dependence: Doctoring in Physical Rehabilitation Practice. *Science, Technology & Human Values*, 34, 55-76.

Struhkamp, R. (2004) *Dealing with disability. Inquiries into a clinical craft*. PhD thesis Amsterdam.

Suchman, L.A. (2007) *Human-machine reconfigurations. Plans and situated actions*. Cambridge University Press.

Suyata, V. (2009) The patient as a knower. Principle and Practice in Siddha Medicine. *Economic and Political Weekly*, XLIV, 16, 76-82.

Taylor, J. (2010) On Recognition, Caring, and Dementia. In: Mol, A., Moser, I. & Pols, J. (eds) *Care in practice. On tinkering in clinics, homes and farms*. Bielefeld: Transcript Verlag, 27-56.

Thygesen, H. (2009) Technology and good dementia care. A study of technology and ethics in everyday care practice. Centre for Technology, Innovation and Culture (TIK), University of Oslo, Phd thesis.

Thygesen, H. & Moser, I. (2010) Technology and good dementia care: an argument for an ethics-in-practice approach. Schillmeier, M. and Domènech, M. (eds.) *New Technologies and Emerging Spaces of Care*. Farnham: Ashgate, 129-147.

Timmermans, S. and M. Berg (2003) *The gold standard: The challenge of evidence-based medicine and standardization in health care*. Philadelphia, PA: Temple University Press.

Timmermans, S., Bowker, G.C. & Star, S.L. (1998) The architecture of difference: Visibility, Control and Comparability in Building a Nursing Interventions Classification. In A. Mol & M. Berg (eds). *Differences in Medicine. Unraveling practices, Techniques and Bodies*. Durham & London: Duke University Press, 202-25.

Tjalsma, D (2007) Remote control! Toekomst en betekenis van telemedicine voor de zorggebruiker (Future and meaning of telemedicine for health care users) Utrecht: NPCF.

Toulmin, S. (1976) On the nature of the physician's understanding. *The journal of medicine and philosophy*, 1, 1, 32-50.

Trappenburg, M. (2008) *Genoeg is genoeg. Over gezondheidszorg en democratie*. Amsterdam: Amsterdam University Press.

Tronto, J. (1993) *Moral boundaries: A political argument for an ethic of care*, New York: Routledge.

Tuckett, A.G. (2002) An ethic of the fitting: a conceptual framework for nursing practice. *Nursing Inquiry*, 5,4 220-227.

Turkle, S. (1984) The second self. Computers and the human spirit. Cambridge, MA: MIT Press.

Velpry, L.(2008) The Patient's View: Issues of Theory and Practice. *Culture, Medicine & Psychiatry*, 32, 238-58.

Verbeek, P.P. (2009), 'Ambient Intelligence and Persuasive Technology: The Blurring Boundaries Between Human and Technology'. *Nanoethics*, 3, 231-242.

Verbeek, P.P. (2006) Materializing Morality. Design ethics and technological mediation. *Science, Technology & Human Values*, 31, 361-80.

Wakefield, B.J., Holaman, J.E., Ray, A. Morse, J., Kienzle, M.G. (2004) Nurse and patient communication via low and high-bandwidth home telecare systems. *Journal of Telemedicine and Telecare*, 10, 156-9.

Webster, A. (2002) Innovative Health technologies and the social: redefining health. Medicine and the Body. *Current Sociology*, 50, 443-57.

Weindling, P. (1989) *Health, Race and German Politics between National Unification and Nazism, 1870-1945*. Cambridge: Cambridge University press.

Whelan, E. (2007) 'No one agrees except for those of us who have it': endometriosis patients as an epistemological community. *Sociology of Health & Illness*, 29, 7, 957-82.

WHO (1998) WHO definition of palliative care. Geneva: WHO.

Willems, D. (2010) Varieties of goodness in high-tech home care. In: Mol, A., Moser, I. & Pols, J. (eds) *Care in practice. On tinkering in clinics, homes and farms*. Bielefeld: Transcript Verlag, 257-76.

Willems, D. et al.(2006) Patient work in end-stage heartfailure. A prospective longitudinal multiple case study. *Palliative Medicine*, 20, 25-33.

Willems D. (2004) Geavanceerde thuiszorgtechnologie: morele vragen bij een ethisch ideaal. (Advanced homecare technology: moral questions with an ethical ideal.) In: *Signalering Ethiek en Gezondheid*, Den Haag: Gezondheidsraad.

Willems, D.L. (2003) Een wereld van verschil. Pluralisme in de medische ethiek. (A world of difference. Pluralism in medical ethics). Inaugural lecture. Amsterdam: Amsterdam University Press.

Willems, D. (2000) Managing one's body using self-management techniques: practicing autonomy. *Theoretical Medicine and Bioethics*, 21, 23-8.

Willems, D. (1995) Tools of Care? Explorations into the Semiotics of Medical Technology. Maastricht University

Willems, D. (1992) Susan's Breathlessness. The construction of professionals and lay persons. In: Lachmund, J. & G. Stollberg (eds) *The social construction of illness*. Stuttgart: Franz Steiner, 105-14.

Wilson, E. (2005) 'Can you think what I feel? Can you feel what I think?' Notes on affect, embodiment and intersubjectivity. AI. *Scandinavian Journal of Media Arts*, 2, 2. http://scan.net.au/scan/journal/display.php?journal id=54.

Winance, M. (2010) Care and disability. Practices of experimenting, tinkering with, and arranging people and technical aids. In: Mol, A.Moser, I. & Pols, J. (eds) *Care in practice. On tinkering in clinics, homes and farms*. Bielefeld: Transcript verlag, 93-118.

Winance, M. (2006) Trying out the wheelchair: The mutual shaping of people and devices through adjustment. *Science, Technology, & Human Values*, 31, 1, 52-72.

Winance M. (2007), Being normally different? Changes to normalisation processes: from alignment to work on the norm, *Disability and Society*, 22, 6, 625-638.

Winance, M. (2001). Thèse et Prothèse. Le processus d'habilitation comme fabrication de la personne. Paris: ENSMP, CSI.

Wittgenstein L. (1953). *Philosophical investigations/Philosophische Untersuchungen*. Oxford: Blackwell.

Wyatt, S. 2008 Technological determinism is dead: Long live technological determinism. In: E.J. Hackett et al. (eds) *The handbook of science and technology studies*. Cambridge: MIT Press, 165-80.

Zola, I.K. (1991) Bringing our bodies and ourselves back in: Reflections on a past, present and future 'medical sociology'. *Journal of Health and Social Behavior*, 32, 1-16.

Zuiderent-Jerak, T. & Van der Grinten, T. (2009) Zorg voor medische technologie. Over het ontwikkelen van zorgtechnologie, vormgeven van technologiebeleid en behartigen van publieke belangen. In: Asveld, L. & Besters, M. (eds) *Medische technologie. Ook geschikt voor thuisgebruik.* (Medical Technology: Also Fit for the home). Den Haag: Rathenau Instituut.

Index of names

Index of subjects

INDEX OF SUBJECTS